Spiked Up

Ready to Run

Unconventional, Myth-Busting,
Scientific, & Proven Training for Runners

Steve D. Sherer

Spiked Up, Ready to Run

Copyright © 2009 Steve D. Sherer

ISBN: 978-1-935125-45-7

Photography by Bob Elliot and Jerry Banks
Front Cover Design by Jerry Banks
Edited by Colleen Duffy

This book is printed in the United States of America
and available for World Wide distribution

To purchase additional copies of this book go to:
www.rp–author.com/Sherer

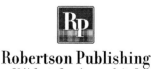

Robertson Publishing
59 N. Santa Cruz Avenue, Suite B
Los Gatos, California 95030 USA
(888) 354-5957 • www.RobertsonPublishing.com

Caution

Certain sections of this book address health, fitness, and medical-related issues like injuries and nutrition for informational purposes only, and should not be construed as medical advice. Please note that such information is not intended to create any physician-patient relationship or supplant any in-person medical consultation or examination. Proper medical attention should always be sought for specific ailments. The following content is not intended to replace proper medical care. Anyone beginning a running program should consult their doctor, especially those over the age of 45, have a family history of coronary disease, or have any other risk factors including high blood pressure, high cholesterol levels, diabetes, obesity, or cigarette smoking.

Dedication

I dedicate this book to my Beautiful Wife Kelsea; her love and patience have spurred me on to greatness since the day I met her. I am eternally grateful for all that you are and will never stop loving you.

To my Mom and Dad that have always been there to support, encourage, and guide me throughout my life. Thank you for being there when I needed you the most and when I didn't.

To my High School coaches Tom Fredrick and David Medley. Your knowledge and encouragement made me believe in myself during the most difficult part of my life. So much so that after years of disappointment and failure I knew there was something more there. And my 'post team' coaches Ed Burke and Willie Harmatz. Thank you for your knowledge and inspiration to help me find my passion once more in a bleak time.

To my college mentor Phil Gillespie. Thank you for helping me see running for what it was and keeping me grounded.

To my great friends all over the world. Thank you... a thousand times, thank you!

Acknowledgements

My special thanks to my good friend Kevin Elliot for his critique and knowledge. Without learning how to lift from you and your connections this book and my career would have never happened.

Thank you Jerry Banks, for your help and encouragement throughout the process of creating this book.

Also, thank you New York Athletic Club for your financial belief in me. Without your help I wouldn't be able to have nearly as many opportunities as I do now.

And finally, my special thanks to Ray Flynn, Brad Yewer, and Susan at Flynn Sports Management. Thank you for helping with my running career as much as you do, you have been a huge help and are greatly appreciated!

Contents

Foreword

By Kevin Elliot

Steve Sherer's running career is a story that has and will continue to inspire other runners to break out of their monotonous training regiments and create a system that is best suited for their unique needs and goals. He has researched, experimented, and proven that his technique of reaching maximal potential will work. Steve's training methods have helped many other runners with whom he has shared his story and techniques.

Steve and I lived and trained together in Los Gatos, CA. During that time, I witnessed the evolution of his mindset and his training. His quest for knowledge and desire to self-train was apparent with many of his out-of-the-box tactics and persistent questions he asked of coaches who tried to change either running style and training methods. From the outset, I could see Steve plotted his own course and was determined to be in charge of the path he would follow.

Not only does the "Shererious" Steve share the secrets of his running methods in *Spiked Up, Ready to Run*; throughout the following pages he also teaches us how to develop as a whole person, finding joy in running as one of life's many activities. Too often athletes fade away and give up their sport due to feelings of failure, a fear of not being good enough, or other negative emotions. Steve addresses these issues by supplying personal examples and detailed instructions on how to cope with these feelings and fears.

As Steve shares his journey of faith and heartache, he proves it is through his trials, triumphs, and failures that his philosophy of ideal training was created. This nationally ranked runner takes us on a journey, which embodies the personality and attitude it takes to become an accomplished track and field athlete as well as a healthy, successful, and confident individual.

Spiked Up, Ready to Run is an effective tool to help runners expand their knowledge and open their minds to change within their lives as well as their training techniques. It is Steve's belief that change can be a powerful motivator to help individuals achieve even greater success. As you read his story, readers are encouraged to keep an open mind to a new way of thinking as they consider the path they have chosen. The methods of training, dieting, strength, conditioning, stretching, and performance Steve endorses are beneficial for all levels and ages of runners who want to hit their maxi-mum potential. It is through his life story and experiences he shares what each of us can do to enhance our athletic training and develop a healthy attitude towards life.

Introduction

Day in the Life

Wake up. A strange room. A strange feeling... race day. Just about everything is different on the day of big races. Everything matters, but nothing is important. You feel like you should do something to get ready for the big race, but there's nothing you can do. Zoning out to the simplest show, like the stand-up comedian I chose to watch one particularly monumental afternoon, can become an emotional roller coaster. Have you ever been close to tears from watching a stand-up comedian perform on T.V.? And that's not because he's ridiculously funny but because you can totally relate with the sad story he tells before delivering the punch line. If you have, either you're incredibly empathetic or you can relate to the case of nerves a runner gets before a big race.

That's where I was, sitting on my bed, curtains closed, Jell-O in my legs, butterflies in my stomach, and attempting to hold back emotional tears while watching stand-up comedy. I had been waiting all day to start warming up for the biggest race of my life to date: the 1500 Semi-Finals of the 2008 Olympic Trials.

The day before, I cruised through the prelims (first of three trials), but encountered a very race savvy group of elite runners in my heat for the Semifinals. I was up against Rob Myers who placed third at the 2004 Olympic Trials, as well as first in the indoor mile at Nationals. My heat also included Bernard Lagat, who is currently the second fastest 1500 meter runner of all time, a gold medalist in the 2007 World Championships in Tokyo, silver medalist in 2004 Olympics, as well as the American record holder in the indoor mile, 1500, 3K, and 5K.

Another contender was David Krummenacker who ran 1:43 in the 800 meter, 3:31 in the 1500 meter, and held many championship racing titles to his name. I was also racing against Alan Webb, the American Mile record holder with a 3:46; he also ran a 3:30 for the 1500; both in 2007, the fastest 1500 meter and mile time in the world that year.

Everybody else in the race came with a good amount of big-race experience, but looking at the heat sheet online, the names of those four runners specifically stuck out. The nervous excitement continued to build as race time approached.

Brushing back the tears from the last stand-up comedian, I finally laced up my shoes and got ready to go warm-up. The drive to the track is always a rush of adrenaline. My dad drove me to the race site, Hayward Field at the University of Oregon in Eugene, Oregon. I wanted to talk to him, and show my appreciation for his support, but the nerves prevented all forms of small talk.

Once I finally entered into the athlete 'corral,' (place we all sit and chill till we warm up) I felt a little more at peace. I was more comfortable being at the track than thinking about the track from my hotel room. I sat there and listened to music while getting excited to warm-up.

About 45 minutes before the race, I decided to start trotting around. Some of the athletes warmed up over an hour before the event, most started about the time I did. I like to stay within sight of the track; I feel more comfortable, so I slowly ran laps around the 200-meter tennis court track behind Hayward Field.

As I passed the other athletes, some were in my race and others were not, I initially gestured hello but that got old after the first time so I stopped. It's always sort of awkward to say hello six or seven times in 12 minutes. Primarily, I tried to focus on the race on my warm-up, although, with a million different ways it could play out, I couldn't decide exactly what to do. This is where I embrace the nerves, and try to feed off of them instead of allowing them consume me. I like to put myself on the starting line and visualize the gun go off, and that is exactly what I did. In my head, I saw the gun go off and felt the jolt of adrenaline that comes with it. I watched the race play out, pictured myself where I wanted to be around the track, imagined the actual feeling of the race, and all the while, I visualized myself relaxed and breathing deeply. Here is where my ability to stay relaxed and focused is key; if I were to lose focus for a second in the race, I would tie up in the lungs first.

The race staff called us all over to the tent. The tent is where they put all the racers before the race; you're thrown together with all of your soon-to-be-competition. We all know each other, but the small talk was just not there. We barely looked at one another as we prepared for the race. I caught a few runners yawning, and I yawned a few times myself. Sometimes when you're nervous, you forget to breathe deeply, so your body does it for you... mine did. It was a serious yawn; I almost snapped a jaw. I tried to keep breathing deep, but nerves can make the most basic task seem strenuous.

They took us to the loading tank under the spectator bleachers. They keep the athletes here for a couple minutes before they go out on the track; there is an 80-meter stretch of track to do strides on. It's very cool to hear the crowd roar from above as if you're about to go on stage; I felt like a gladiator.

From there, the official took us onto to the University of Oregon's Hayward Field track surrounded by an enthusiastic crowd. Eugene, Oregon, is otherwise referred to as Track Town, USA and Hayward Field track has seen a fair amount of history on it. The famous Steve Prefontaine movies were filmed on it, and the best of the best have raced on it. Walking onto this track was such an awesome feeling. The excitement of the very knowledgeable track crowd was palpable and started to pick up as we entered the track. Game time.

We all did a few last-minute sprint drills and a couple of strides on the backstretch as the race staff hyped us up over the loud speaker. I never know what to do when they announce my name in front of a crowded stadium. Big-game introduction training isn't part of a runner's focus. I remembered my former roommate Nick Willis (who earned the 1500 meter silver medal at in the 2008 Olympics) would always give a simple wave to the crowd, so that's what I did. It worked. I didn't feel like an idiot. We all lined up and did our little leg shake-out things. Before I knew it, the starter had the gun up. BANG! We were off.

At last! The beautiful sound of the gun; this point in race day is actually the least nerve-racking part, believe it or not. No more thinking about the race, just doing it. It was a clean start; Webb took off and grabbed the lead with Lagat on his tail. I grabbed some rail right away and just tried to relax. This is the furthest inside point going around the track, so you run less distance, but can get in a box or shoved to the back easily. I always seem to get passed and end up in the back of the pack, and that's where I was... dead last.

My goal was to finish in the top six so I could qualify for the finals without spending too much energy. That's the key in these major events with qualifiers, and semi-finals before the finals. Keep moving forward, while still leaving something in the tank for the next round. It gets more difficult in the semi-finals when you have the caliber of runners I was facing in that race.

I was okay with my last-place position, going with the "it doesn't matter where you start, but where you finish" ideology. It was nice being back there out of trouble as we ran around the track. I could see the race unfold and then at the right time planned to make a critical move to get to the front. My legs felt great at the end of the first lap so I just stayed relaxed and enjoyed the moment. The second lap was uneventful. My legs weren't tightening up and my breathing was solid. The crowd started to pick up, along with my adrenaline. It was time to get to the front.

I made my move at around 800 meters into the race on the backstretch. I quickly went from last to the front. I hopped right on Webb's shoulder, who was leading at the time, just as we entered the curve from the back stretch. As soon as he felt me there he picked it up and I went with him. This created a gap between him and Lagat. I grabbed some more rail between them as we had entered the curve, which put me in perfect position going into the last lap. I still felt like I had another move left in me, so I was pretty confident at this point. However, my breathing was a bit heavier so I wasn't in the clear; in a race like this, anything can happen.

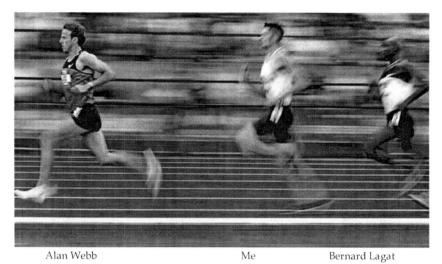

Alan Webb   Me   Bernard Lagat

Photo by: *Bob Elliott, The Athletic Connection*

We held those positions coming out of the turn while racing down the straightaway. As we headed into the last lap, the crowd really picked it up and began to roar. I was in great position and feeling pretty good going into that last lap. I decided to hang on Webb's shoulder until I had to make a move; the last 100 meters of championship races are always a toss up when everybody has a kick. I stayed there as long as possible, patiently waiting for the inevitable. I just had to get one of the top six places to move on to the finals, but these runners were not going to give it to me without a fight.

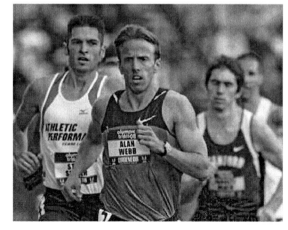

Photo by: *Bob Elliott, The Athletic Connection*

At about 150 meters to go, heading into the home stretch Myers made his move. He took off and passed me and Webb. Knowing this would happen, I had put myself on Webb's outside shoulder so I didn't get boxed in behind him. Luckily, it worked; I had enough room to move out right behind Myers. We moved around Webb and took off to the finish line. Myers has a very fast last 100 meters if he's feeling good, and he was. I just stayed right behind him.

It was thrilling to be running fast, closing in on the finish line in second place with the entire stadium, a sold-out crowd of 21,000 track fans in the legendary Hayward field, screaming their heads off. Crazy. I figured I was clearly in so I just stayed right behind Myers through the line. In the last 10 meters Lagat jumped out in front and Leer moved up right beside me, just in front of Webb. I made it! I was going to the finals!

The crowd was out of control, still screaming as we jogged off the track. It seemed surreal, perhaps due to the oxygen debt to the brain or my newfound ability to compete with the best. I did have some junk in my legs because the last 100 meters was an all-out sprint, but the hype of getting into the finals helped it dissipate quickly. This was the furthest I had ever made it in an outdoor national event!

The Finals

Unfortunately, the Finals for the 2008 Olympic Trials did not go as well as the prelims. As soon as the gun went off, I got caught up in the main pack. There was so much pushing and shoving going on in the pack; it kept me from relaxing so I did not have my normal great last 500 meters. I did experience difficulty breathing because my asthma decided to remind me of its presence for the first time in two years and kicked into full gear. Along with the bumping, and being out of position, the stress of the finals probably helped trigger the asthma.

I did learn more about myself and what I require in order to race better, but I was still disappointed. I knew my fitness level was there to make the team, but poor race strategies kept me out of the games. In 2012, however, I'll be going for a "spot of tea" next to Big Ben.

I have not always been the athlete who could cruise into the finals of the Olympic Trials like this. Before embarking on my own search for the holy grail of training protocol, I, too, fell victim to traditional training methods, and the inevitable results: slow racing and burnout.

Improving Times

It's been a long, hard road with many ups and downs in my training. I almost stopped running three times before the finals because I thought I would never run as fast as I thought I could run. I guess I still haven't, but who has? What I have done is devised a workout plan that has taken me from 3:45.99 minutes to 3:36.81 minutes in the 1500 meter; from 1:52.6 to 1:47.7 in the 800 meter; and from 4:01.8 to 3:56.00 in the mile. All of these time improvements took place in less than two years of coaching myself and using a non-traditional and unorthodox training system.

What's Your Secret?

With the many training questions thrown at me, I feel that the methods I used to get results are probably something other people would like to learn as well. Many people ask me, "What's your secret?" My secret is simple really; it's my training. Finding the perfect training system, or rather, the perfect system for me, has allowed me to improve my fitness level and race faster.

Sometimes I find myself thinking the common thought: "if only I knew then what I know now", referring to my college running career. I wish I had the current training knowledge I now possess. I wish I had known how to stay injury free in the weight room. I wish I had known the right amount of time to push a base run or not to push a base run. I wish I knew stability shoes cause injuries. I didn't, but I do now. This is my gift to you, the running athlete. Now you will know, and in the words of G.I. Joe: "knowing is half the battle."

I think this type of training is a much-needed variation from our current mid- to long-distance training protocol. Considering how awful we do against other countries in the Olympics and other world championships, one would think we would start trying something new! Here is a "something new" our current training style desperately needs.

Navigating the Lanes

I wrote Section 1, the The Science section, during my 2008 season right after I ran a 3:56 minute indoor mile; the fourth fastest first time under 4-minute mile ever run by an American. I was really excited about the training so I had to write it down. I continued with the same training all the way until August, where I ran at the Hershey Track and Field meet in Philadelphia and called it a season. I did not switch up the training much at all through that entire time, except when I sprained my knee when I tripped over a gopher hole two months before the Olympic Trials. However, after I was fully recovered, I was able to continue the same training again to run my 3:36.8 minute in June.

If you want to get to know me, hear some funny stories about what I've been through, and see how my running career has progressed, I put Section 2 My Story in there for you. It's a valuable section for a runner and a coach since I wrote it after my season when I had learned a little more about racing after my 3:56 minute mile; and because it's a fun runner's story.

Section 1:

The Science

Introduction:

Well, it's been a long road, but I have enjoyed the journey that has taken me to where I am today. I wrote this book because I feel I have accrued a good amount of running-related knowledge to offer the running world. I have experienced many different types of training and have researched a great deal of information to get myself into the shape I am in. This book is an overview of all the different training tactics I have read about and tried out during the past three years of coaching myself.

I have had some great training experiences, and some "learning" training experiences. In this section, I will try and take you through and summarize the various research I have conducted, as well as the books and fitness articles I have read. I also elaborate on different track coach gurus, weight-lifting experts, along with professional athletes and elite runners I have had the pleasure of talking to and discussing training with; and the different thought processes I have put into my training program. It is a never-ending journey, but I do feel that what I have now is a very effective and, according to some, unconventional training program that I have proven and still am using to great success.

Using this program I improved my personal best in the mile from a 4:01.8 mile to later running a 3:56.0 indoor mile. I also improved from a conventionally trained and earned 3:45.99 in the 1500-meter race to a 3:36.8 using my self-developed methodology.

This new approach to training is what I have to offer the coaches and athletes who are reading this book. Perhaps not everyone will improve as much as I have and perhaps some will improve more. Not all runners react to the same training regimen in the same way. I just know that it has worked wonders for me and is of great benefit to those I am coaching.

Read it with an open and analytical mind. Take my thoughts and ideas and integrate them with your own personal experience to develop an optimal workout for you or those you are coaching. Use what you want to use and don't use what you don't want to. The best training is optimized for each runner, so be mindful of your strengths and let me help you build on them.

Thank you for taking the time to read my thoughts and ideas on perfecting a training program for you and/or your runners. I know you will get something useful out of this book that will make you and/or your runners faster... in some cases, crazy fast.

For all the coaches out there:

Dear Coach,

You are an amazing person and are changing the lives of countless young people in a positive way. I really do appreciate coaches; after all, I am a coach. But seriously, what you do is great for the community and your athletes.

I have had some amazing coaches myself and learned from them. I've also endured some less than great coaches whose biggest problem was that they felt the need to put on a front of infallibility who believe what they do is the best and only way to train. This type is not willing to listen to athletes' suggestions about what might work best for them. One of the best things a coach can learn is that they do not know everything in the coaching/running world. Get over it; no one does, and in fact, no one can. Throughout a good coaches their career they will never stop learning new things about training. With this mindset, a coach can look to improve their athletes' training and build a better training program every year.

In this section, I will try to shed some light on blind spots that coaches might have. Coaches must deal with all types of athletes: those who hate to do any hard work and find any excuse possible to avoid a hard workout or the super-motivated athlete, for example. Basically, every runner is different.

In coaching there are VERY few certainties. A coach will have one person adapt very well to a training program and get faster, while another runner on the same training program might not improve or may even get slower. A coach will see some people get injured every week, others get sick, and yet other athletes can jump off of cliffs, run barefoot on cement, be a charter member in a local fight club, and never even get the sniffles.

Throughout this section, I will not cover every single way to coach or to train an athlete. No single book can or should even try. But I will try to elaborate on what seems to be misplaced in today's running world. This is a good tool for coaches or if you're self-coaching because it will give you more options in your arsenal to coach different types of athletes. Have you ever had an athlete who shows flashes of speed but lacks the endurance to match? No matter how many long runs, or long intervals or traditional tempo runs you put him/her through, he/she cannot seem to put that speed to good use in a race? Then this book may provide just the right tool to help that runner breakout and achieve great things.

I will also go over one of the most important tools to making a runner faster: staying injury free. If a runner cannot train, he or she will not get better, and odds are, he or she will get worse. I personally do not believe in "rebuilding years" or whatever coaches often refer to seasons in which athletes do not improve. If an athlete does not get better, it's time to recheck the training because that's what it all comes down to, training.

For all of the athletes:

Dear Athlete,

You rock. Keep trying to do your best and stay passionate about each aspect of your life you consider important. I assume you are passionate about running if you are reading this book. Passion is a key ingredient for anyone who wants to excel.

One thing you should realize is that you do not know everything there is to know in the running world. Odds are, coaches will know a fair amount more than you about running; coaches also have more experience in seeing what works for runners; and they have done more research than you have regarding what works.

However, athletes who know the most about their sport are generally the best in their sport. They know their bodies and what's necessary to work well. Athletes also understand what works for them and what doesn't work (especially what doesn't). The more knowledge you gain, the better you can possibly be. You do not have to reinvent the wheel; there are tons of different types of athletes who have tried various techniques to attain optimum fitness and excel at their sport! Learn from them; keep increasing your knowledge as much as you can.

There are millions of great resources available to you: the Internet, talking with elite runners or coaches, talking training with elite people in other sports, resources at the library, magazines, and journal articles. It's also important to assess yourself as you continue in the sport. Life is a never-ending learning experience; the day you stop learning is the day you die. "My people die because lack of knowledge," Hosea 4:6. My advice to you is don't allow yourself to die; it's a choice. Keep learning, and keep working.

Being heavily involved in the running world, I seem to hear the same things from different people over and over again. Most of the time I hear a type of catch phrase that a runner or coach says to themselves or their athlete that sounds good, until you think about it and find it stupid. Some of these axioms can have a little truth, but generally they just sound much better than they really are, masking the real problem. They can also create beliefs that are quite negative to the runner as well. Because of these commonly held beliefs in the running world that cause more harm than benefit, I am compelled to dispel a few myths that stand out to me the most.

Myth to Athletes #1:

"Running is 90% Mental and 10% Physical"... BAH!

I hear coaches and runners say that running is "90% mental and only 10% physical (or more mental than physical)." Throw that idea out the window, with passion. During competition, running, similar to most sports, is 95% physical and 5% mental.

If you've trained your body to move faster, react quicker, push harder, breathe easier, relax easier, and absorb more oxygen than your competitors, then you're going to win 95% of the time, even if you are a blithering idiot. Of course, you have to run fast and be able to turn left, make sure you don't go out way too quickly, and try not to run into people; all of that comes with practice. The time to think is during training; the time to "just do it" is in competition.

The common phrase after a bad race is: "I guess you/I didn't want it bad enough." Or similarly: "You/I just didn't compete!" I'm pretty sure competitive runners never go to the line and decide to run slow, shoot for last place, and maybe get a few pity claps for finishing. People want to win and saying they do not will probably make them win less. Figuring out how to get runners in shape to win more will help them do exactly that, win more.

In one of my favorite quotes William James says: "We do not sing because we are happy, we are happy because we sing!" I have to agree with him. Try smiling in the mirror. Go on, do it now. The bigger the grin, the happier you feel. I normally just start laughing, especially if I'm with another person. Just stand next to somebody looking in the mirror, put a huge goofy grin on your face, and see what happens. Or sing your favorite song, unless you have an awful voice. Whistle instead. Just kidding! Sing anyways. Pretty soon you'll find yourself in a much better mood than when you started.

You have much more control over your emotions and than you may realize; your actions can change your feelings.

The best way to build your confidence and bring your head game along as well is to train your body to handle the workload and see yourself getting fitter. However, training does take passion, discipline, and drive to do it well; this could be considered a mental part of running.

I remember reading about the Law of Cognitive Dissonance in my Psychology Class back in College; this is when your feelings/beliefs don't meet up with your actions so there is disarray in your brain. The opposite is consonance, where your feelings and actions meet up in harmony, so your brain is tranquil. Basically, the more you put into something and work towards something without any external rewards, the more you force yourself to internally enjoy it. If it's a means to an end, you will not like it. If it's an end in itself, you'll love it. (If I was a marriage counselor and I heard the all to common, "I just don't love him/her anymore." I would tell them, "So you're basically telling me that you don't do anything for them at all anymore without expecting something in return, because if you did things for him just to do it, you would be forced to love him/her.) For running, if you look at it as a way to get money, better at another sport, look good, get a better butt, or any other reason that just enjoying it for what it is… you inevitably won't like it. This is probably why turning the sport into a profession has ruined it for many athletes. Once you're getting paid to do it, it loses some of its intrinsic value. Do it for the pure joy of doing it and it will always be enjoyable. Like when you were a kid and you just wanted to race your buddy to the playground so you both went all out and probably liked it. Start making running a means to a end and you will eventually be sick of it.

Do it for the pure joy of 'just doing it'. Good job on the slogan Nike!

I think I've gone down enough rabbit holes on this one… sorry. But do what it takes to increase your passion for the sport. Learn more about it, get better at it, talk to others about it, and do it. You did not feel passion for the sport before you actually did it; passion developed by actually doing it. Like I said before, your mental side will come around with your physical actions.

Myth to Athletes #2

"It can take years to adapt to a different training system"... BAH!

Time is one of your most precious resources. Don't waste it by listening to people say that you need to "be patient and give your body time to adapt to the different training stimulus." The fact of the matter is: <u>if you're not getting faster every year, it's time to change your training</u>. PERIOD. No ifs, ands, or buts. My definition of insanity is doing things the same way and expecting a different result. Apparently this doesn't apply to the running world. When coaches ask you to be patient and wait for the improvement, it could mean one of two things: they really think you'll eventually adapt and might get better (you might... eventually, but not very much and definitely not get as fast as you should or could). Or they might just not want to put in the extra work and time it takes to create a semi-individualized workout program for you.

No matter what the answer, you need to get involved with your own training program. Your coach may be overloaded or may not see that special spark in you that would make it worth his time and effort. If this is the case, shame on your coach for not caring about it when you obviously do. But be sympathetic as well, individualizing and perfecting a program for every athlete would be impossible; even developing an adequate one is a lot of work.

Just talking to a coach about custom programs will generally put them on the defensive about their training. It is not unusual for a coach to interpret your innocent comment: "I think a different type of training will work a little better for me," as: "your training sucks and I hate you." So be careful how you broach the subject because I think I could have had better training discussions with my coaches in the past. Okay, I know I could have had much better ones; the various training talks with a few different coaches resulted in every conversation with lots of anger, yelling, and resentment... not from me, but from them.

In every case I tried to be as cordial as possible, but it's just something that I think the average coach doesn't want to hear from their athlete. Face-to-face is probably the best way to try this. If you are thinking of e-mail, just remember the standard rule with e-mail: if it can be interpreted incorrectly, it will be. I wouldn't leave this to e-mail.

This book will help you discover what type of training you like, and what type of training you don't like. I will go into detail to explain why I train like I do, and very briefly throw out various alternative methods. While I do not advocate them, I know many great runners and coaches alike who do. Either way, improving your training knowledge will increase your confidence in any way you choose to train. And I guarantee, there will be something in this book that you will be able to add to your training routine and benefit greatly.

I once called myself a princess on an online interview with LetsRun.com, and I stand by my word. If there is something in my program that I don't like I will crawl down 100 mattresses to revise it before I can sleep. I advise you to do the same thing.

Volume:
"How Many Miles Do You Run?"

I think the most common question I get from runners and non-runners alike is: "How many miles a week do you run?!?" As if this has a direct relationship to my success as a runner? How many miles you run a week is a very personal, and I think, nonsensical, question. It's similar to asking a successful businessman: "what do you wear to work that makes you earn so much money?!" He could wear a suit, a uniform, a Big Bird costume, overalls, or nothing at all... don't try that last one. Each would possibly end in different results financially. In my opinion, how many miles a runner runs a week is a similar question. There is not a magic number of miles for every runner to make you run at your optimum level.

Running is a high-impact power sport, unlike swimming, biking, and rowing. This means it's much more taxing on the body and you can quickly dig yourself into a hole from it, both physically and mentally. This is why competitive swimmers and bikers can practice their sport for three to six hours daily, and recover quickly enough to do it again the next day.

Runners cannot do this. Every time your foot strikes you are applying at least two G's of pressure (two times the force of gravity) on every single one of you leg joints and bones. Ligaments, tendons, and leg muscles take most of that force as well. For this reason, you have to listen to your body because if you run too much, you will get injured. The moral of the story: don't over do the miles. Other than not running at all, which would be the worst for performance, the best methods I've found to prevent injuries include these three equally important actions: get into the weight room regularly and lift correctly, run only "smart miles" to get you into running shape or recovered, and run in low stability shoes like racing flats for all your runs.

Running puts you through a type of osteoporosis and arthritis, caused by the high impact of the sport, which damages muscles much more quickly. Lifting weights correctly strengthens your muscles, bones, and joints to handle the load and stress of running. I'll go over this in depth in the weight-lifting chapter. Running is the most effective part of your training but it is the hardest on the body. This means you can burnout and overreach pretty easily, but it also gets you in shape in the least amount of time.

To better explain "smart miles," I took it from the common business law of 80/20. I think there was a coach who used the same theory before, but I don't recall which coach. Anyways, for our use, 80% of your fitness is derived from 20% of your workouts, (in business: 80% of income comes from 20% of clients). For me, my high-intensity workouts total around nine miles or less if I include my hill interval workouts, which means I should run around forty miles a week. I don't really keep track of miles or have a weekly mileage goal to hit because I like to decide which workout I'm going to do based on how I feel, not based off of an arbitrary number. These miles have to have a purpose; I'll explain how to make sure you optimize these miles in the *Workouts* section.

Again, the magic number for miles run a week does not exist because everybody will adapt differently to the stress of running. Some runners' joints, muscles, or bones will get messed up if they run over 50 MPW. These are normally the fast adapters, their muscles and joints can wear out a bit more quickly, but they adapt more quickly to a lower volume of stimulus. This does not make them a sprinter by any means. I know some great marathoners that run around 35-50 miles a week and some amazing 5K runners that did the same. But that does mean you have to train them like a sprinter (greyhounds) more often than you do with the distance lovers (huskies) of the running world.

The distance lovers are the runners who physically resemble toothpicks year round. They can run over 100 miles a week using single daily workouts, and take a little bit longer to develop. This craving for miles, however, does not necessarily make them long-distance runners. I know 400 and 800 meter guys who like to get over 90 MPW and do 18-mile runs. These guys don't consider a two miles a run. They make fun of people like me who put on running shoes to run for a several miles and rarely run over five miles at once. I think this is the most natural type of runner, some Utah-Harvard scientists discovered 26 distance running features that make us humans a perfect distance runner in the animal kingdom. Tribes of ancient populations have been known to run down deer and antelope from making them exhausted. And, although we're the most obese nation in the world, it seems like EVERYBODY runs the marathon. Basically, we already know how to run for a long time slow; the trick is to figure out how to run very fast for 2 – 4 minutes.

Why do I run so little mileage in so many runs? Well, I always hated running long distances at once. My body complained bitterly to me and I didn't see great results, but I did it because people told me that it would make me a better runner. Many coaches said: "To be a better runner you have to run more!" It wasn't until I was working as a personal trainer in California that a 1984 Olympic hammer thrower named Ed Burke talked to me about a few studies on testosterone (T) and the human growth hormone (HGH) compared with C-reactive protein (CRP) and cortisol in weight lifters throughout the lifting process. They didn't inject it into them, but they measured the levels of each in the lifters blood at different times while lifting.

- *Cortisol is part of the fight or flight response. When faced with a physically or mentally stressful situation, cortisol increases the flow of glucose (as well as protein and fat) from the body's tissues into the bloodstream in order to increase energy and physical readiness to handle stressful situations or threats. Cortisol is catabol-*

ic and elevated cortisol levels can cause the loss of muscle tissue by facilitating the process of converting lean tissue into glucose, not good when you are trying to strengthen muscles.

- **C-Reactive Protein (CRP)** *is a protein in blood serum involved in inflammatory reactions and general resistance to bacterial infection. If you are sick, injured, going through a lot of stress, inflamed from injuries or not getting enough sleep, this bad boy will show up. It can also be a precursor for coronary heart disease and stroke, as well as Type II Diabetes, which can block insulin, and even psychotic effects like depression. High levels of CRP are found in victims of physical burnout.*

- **Human Growth Hormone (HGH)** *is a powerful anabolic hormone that occurs naturally in the human body. It is produced by the pituitary gland in the brain and stimulates the growth of muscle, cartilage, and bone. It also allows tired muscles to recover quicker, allowing you to train harder and more often.*

- **Testosterone (T)** *is linked to enhanced libido, increased energy, increased production of red blood cells, and protection against osteoporosis. It has also been shown to be responsible for instrumental (social) aggression, which is premeditated behavior used as a means to some non-hostile end (Bushman & Anderson, 2001). Instrumental aggression is the form of aggression commonly associated with competitive sports. Basically it supplies the drive to make you want to get better, work harder, and compete. Once it drops, you lose this drive. Drive it low enough, and for long enough, and you can drive yourself deep into burnout.*

What one of the studies found was a significant increase in T and HGH production for the first 30 minutes of exercise, with a plateau for 15 minutes or so; production then decreased for another 15 minutes until the levels returned back to the beginning levels of T and HGH production. After an hour of a hard workout, athletes can dig themselves into a big hole as both T and HGH (the good stuff that helps you get more fit) fall off dramatically and cortisol will sky rocket.

CRP and cortisol has an inverse relationship with T and HGH. In the study, the levels decreased in the first 30 min of exercise, plateaued for the next 15 minutes, and then started rising for another 15 minutes. At 60 minutes, CRP and cortisol crossed the T and HGH levels, and took off exponentially for each minute thereafter of a hard workout. Basically, at 30 to 45 minutes, T and HGH levels are the highest and CRP and cortisol levels are the lowest. Alternatively, after an hour of hard work, like a long run, CRP and cortisol levels are higher and rising while T and HGH levels plummet.

Now you see the dilemma of long, hard workouts. Testosterone and HGH are anabolic hormones in the body that helps you make physical gains but they fall off dramatically if a workout lasts longer than 45 minutes. With your body under the stress of a long, hard workout, it begins to release cortisol to increase the glucose levels in your blood. This is probably why long distance runners are so skinny with no muscle and typically have low testosterone/estrogen to name a couple. Funny study I had done on accident, I had some random drug tests done on me in 2008 and the only thing they found was a higher than normal amount of testosterone in my urine, but not enough to test positive. I was pretty happy about that. I bet most distance runners couldn't say the same thing.

One of the mechanisms used to produce glucose includes converting it from muscle, this is exactly the opposite of what you want to happen. When glucose is converted from muscle, the good stuff is depleted and the bad stuff is growing in your system exponentially and that is a condition you want to avoid. In addition to eating away at your precious lean muscle mass, high cortisol levels can decrease bone density and cause stress fractures. It may weaken the immune system, reduce libido, and cause insomnia, impotence, amenorrhea, excess sweating, hypertension, proximal muscle weakness (hips, shoulders), hirsutism (facial male-pattern hair growth), and infertility. Patients frequently suffer various psychological disturbances, ranging from euphoria to psychosis. Depression and anxiety are also common. (1) Needless to say, you don't want this stuff floating around in your system too long. When I looked at all the indicators for Over Training Syndrome, I found it interesting that they are all highly correlated with high cortisol level indicators. Coincidence? I think not.

These studies are predominantly conducted on weight lifters because they're the easiest to test, but I think the results are easily comparable to runners. Running is more strenuous on the body than lifting in general and potentially could raise these levels at an even faster rate. I think that if you do go for longer runs, keep an easy pace to help curb the cortisol secretion throughout the longer-duration workouts. But why would you want to waste that much time? You could get better aerobic results going shorter and harder, and you could get active rest and pure recovery just as well going very slow for 10 to 30 minutes.

Another reason I like short bouts of continuous runs and love interval training on the track at goal race pace, or faster, is because I believe it's the best way to increase your highest rate of oxygen consumption or VO2 MAX, thus improving fitness, endurance, speed, and everything else. Darby and Associates (2) came to the same conclusion as a result of their research. When low-moderate intensity long-bout exercise was compared with repeated maximal intensity short-bout exercise on oxygen consumption (VO2), they found:

1. High-intensity exercise, either intermittent or continuous, increases recovery oxygen consumption more than prolonged low intensity exercise. (3, 4)
2. Human growth hormone (somatotropin), an activator of lipolysis and muscle adaptation, is stimulated by the exercise intensity threshold. (5)
3. Plasma glutamine, an essential amino acid for the normal functioning of the immune system, is decreased after endurance events and prolonged exercise (intermittent and continuous), but increased after short-term, high-intensity exercise. (6)
4. The dominant acid extruding system associated with intense exercise is the lactate/H+ co-transporter, shown to increase

its transport capacity in human skeletal muscle with high-intensity exercise training. (7)

5. High-intensity training, but not moderate-intensity training, has been shown to increase both monocarboxylate transporter 1 (MCT) and lactate uptake in skeletal muscle. (8) *(MCT is the mechanism that brings fuel into your mitochondria, which activates your muscles).*

6. Moderate-intensity aerobic training that improves the maximal aerobic power does not change anaerobic capacity, whereas high-intensity intermittent training may improve both anaerobic and aerobic energy supplying systems significantly, probably through imposing intensive stimuli on both systems. (9)

7. Studies examining the interactive effects of intensity, frequency, and duration, have shown that the greatest improvements in aerobic power occur at the greatest intensity. (10)

8. High-intensity interval training (HIIT) is more effective for stimulation of fatty-acid oxidation than continuous sub-maximal exercise training (11) *(While some distance runners may not care that HIIT is more effective at fat loss than moderate-intensity aerobic exercise, it is further proof that the body adapts faster with HIIT. I do, however, know that you can burn a higher percentage of fat for fuel at lower intensities. That doesn't refute this point; it simply shows less of a need for glycogen stores at very low intensities. A great way to melt fat off is HIIT and followed with low-intensity long- duration running. I'll go over that later.)*

9. Human growth hormone, stimulated by the exercise intensity threshold (12) was found to increase in supra-maximal shorter intervals, but not in longer, higher-intensity intervals; cortisol levels sky rocketed in the longer intervals. *(Personally, I hate running at high intensities over 400 meters, so my body agrees with this finding.)*

This is the scientific reasoning behind my dislike for runs that exceed 30 minutes at a steady pace. From a personal perspective, I run for two or four minutes for my race, so why would I need to run for 45 minutes or longer? And every time my various past coaches made me run a long run, which I immensely disliked, my body would tie up more and more by the second. I have a biological clock that kicks me in the hamstring every second after hour-long runs. I just don't enjoy it and can't make my body adapt to it. While there are some days I feel better than others doing longer runs, I never really enjoyed running that long, which brings me to my third HUGE myth.

Myth to Athletes #3:

"Work on you weaknesses and you'll run faster"

This statement is true, but not the way runners typically understand it. It sounds so good and wise, it's easy to believe it, but I think the statement has ruined many good runners. Coaches and runners use this advice to say something to the extent, "if you're not good at long intervals/hills/sprints/long runs, you should focus on that until you improve and enjoy it. Then you will race faster." I always heard college coaches and runners say something similar to this: "He ran a (pick your race) in (pick your time), running only 35 miles a week. Imagine how good he would be if he ran double that!" BAH! If it's working for the runner, keep it going. When improvement tapers off, then it is time to reevaluate the training.

You are a unique human being who functions differently than everybody else. If you are one of those runners who loves running tons of miles, long intervals, high volume, and can't put on your shoes and run less than seven miles at once, keep doing it. Your speed will come around and race times will go down with the training stimulus you enjoy. Likewise, if you're like me and you hate long intervals on the track, dislike running over six miles, never run a long run, and love speed, do that! Endurance will increase and your times will get faster. The key is to avoid giving yourself bad stimulus, the wrong training processes, that your body doesn't handle well; instead of helping your weakness, you mainly harm your strength.

If running is too much of a mental stress, you'll eventually hate it and rarely ever improve. Running should be enjoyable; you should be excited and maybe a bit nervous about the workout, but not terrified of it. You shouldn't finish with a base run feeling like you just got in a fight and lost. Listen to your body, it knows best. And most importantly, enjoy and feel confident in your training, but always try to improve upon it.

Once after a long-interval workout with moderately high intensities (Which I enjoy even less than a long run) I was laying in bed with my whole body pulsating at 70 beats per minute (BPM) right along with my heart at 3 A.M. in the morning. Now for some people, 70 BPM may not be alarming but I have a resting heart rate around 30 and feeling it pound away at 40 beats above normal while in bed is far from normal. I'm pretty sure that feeling my whole body pulsate right along with it was not a good sign either.

Needless to say, I think my body did not like the long repeats and I know it mentally destroyed me. I was scared to run another workout that was remotely similar to that one. This is typically the case with all types of workouts I detest. They don't do much for me and end up being more of a stressor to my mind and body than a confidence boost and performance enhancer. Let your strengths help your weaknesses, but always try to focus on your strengths.

A non-scientific rationale for my type of training comes from the only man in history to win the three distance races in a single Olympics; he won the 5K, 10K, and the marathon in the 1952 Helsinki Olympic Games. The Czechoslovakian runner Emil Zatopek not only won, but set Olympic records in all three events. Later that year, he held every world record from the 10K to the marathon, and in 1954, he earned the world record for the 5K.

Zatopek summed it up very nicely when he said: "When I was young, I was too slow. I thought, why should I practice running slow? I already know how to run slow… I must learn to run fast by practicing to run fast. So I ran 100 meter very fast. People said, "Emil, you are crazy. You are training to be a sprinter. You have no chance." I said, "Yes, but if I run 100 meters 20 times, that is 2 kilometers and that is no longer a sprint." "

Zatopek took his training ideas from the great Paavo Nurmi, who holds *Time Magazine's* title of Greatest Olympian of All Time. *Time* no doubt awarded the Finnish runner with this honor because he competed in three Olympic games, won nine medals, set 33 world records, and didn't lose any of the 80 cross country races he ran in his life. He also coached the Finnish running team for the 1936 Berlin Olympics. In those games, his runners won 14 Olympic medals, capturing all three of the 10K medals. Zatopek said this about Nurmi and the intervals methods he learned from him: "I never spoke with Paavo Nurmi, but running is easily understandable. You must be fast enough and you must have endurance. So, you run fast enough for speed and repeat it many times for endurance." One word: BRILLIANT!!

Of course, the best reasoning for quality over quantity is from one of my track heroes, the first of the self-coached milers, Rodger Banister. This lunchtime miler completed most of his training in 30 minutes or less and is considered to have the greatest sports accomplishment of all time. His 10 x 400 meter workout and variations of it will probably go down in history as the best miler workout of all time. His volume could not have been very high per week if he only had 30 minutes a day to train.

I think the best answer for the frequently asked question: "How many miles should I run?" is: "I don't know." I don't. It is up to you and what you are excited and motivated to do. Knowing what you like to do for training, keeping training based on the races you want to compete in and running far enough and fast enough for speed endurance is a good non-specific, scientifically based answer. So like the philosophers of old said, "know thyself," or a little harshly put: "the unexamined life is not worth living." Don't let others dictate your future. Own up, take responsibility, and find out what's best for you.

1. Raff H, Findling JW. "*A physiologic approach to diagnosis of the Cushing's syndrome.*" Ann Intern Med 2003;138:980-91.

2. Darby M, Smith MJ, Melby C^s, Gotshall R. *"Comparison on the Effect of Long-Bout Exercise with Repeat Short-Bout Exercise on Oxygen Consumption"* Departments of Exercise & Sport Science and Food Science and Human Nutrition CSU, Fort Collins CO. (1998)

3. Brockman, L. et al. *"Oxygen uptake during recovery from intense intermittent running and prolonged walking."* J. Sports Med. Phys. Fitness. 1993; 33(4): 330-336.

4. Laforgia J. et al. *"Comparison of energy expenditure elevations after submaximal and supramaximal running."* J. Appl. Physiol. 1997; 82(2): 661-666.

5. Snegovskaya V et al. *"Steroid and pituitary hormone responses to rowing: relative significance of exercise intensity and duration and performance level."* Eur. J. Appl. Physiol. 1993; 67(1): 59-65.

6. Parry-Billings M et al. *"Plasma amino acid concentrations in the overtraining syndrome: possible effects on the immune system."* Med. Sci. Sports Exerc. 1992: 24(12): 1353-1358.

7. Pilegaard H et al. Effect of high-intensity exercise training on lactate/H+ transport capacity in human skeletal muscle. Am. J. Physiol. 1999; 276(2 Pt 1): 255-261.

8. Baker SK et al. *"Training intensity-dependent and tissue -specific increases in lactate uptake and MCT-1 in heart and muscle."* J. Appl. Physiol. 1998; 84(3): 987-994.

9. Tabata, I. et al. *"Effects of moderate-intensity endurance and high-intensity intermittent training on anaerobic capacity and V02 max."* Med. Sci. Sports Exerc. 1996: 28(10): 1327-1330.

10. Wenger HA et al. *"The interactions of intensity, frequency and duration of exercise training in altering cardiorespiratory fitness."* Sports Med. 1986; 3(5):346-356.

11. Chilibeck PD et al. *"Higher mitochondrial fatty acid oxidation following intermittent versus continuous endurance exercise training."* Can. J. Physiol. Pharmacol. 1998; 76(9):891

12. Snegovskaya V et al. *"Steroid and pituitary hormone responses to rowing: relative significance of exercise intensity and duration and performance level."* Eur. J. Applied Physiology 1993; 67(1): 59-65.

Lane 2

Periodization:
When Should I Do Which Type of Workouts?

This is a great question, if you truly want to know the answer, that is. The first thing to realize is you will never fully know the answer to this question, but you can come pretty darn close. There are too many outside variables and internal variables to determine which workouts are best for you and when they're best for you. So I will go over the a few periodization plans: the most common periodization formula in the running world; a variation of that one; and a less commonly known periodization program, my personal favorite, Daily Undulated Periodization.

The Most Common Plan

Periodization is not an unknown thing in the running world. I always hear runners talking about it, especially early in their season: "Well, I'm really happy with my race (slower than PB, but not an awful time) because I've been doing mainly strength lately in preparation for (fill in the blank with a bigger race later one in the year)…" This is the base phase. This is a very distance-oriented phase with a focus on Type I muscle fibers (slow twitch); low-intensity, high-volume work; little to no racing; and includes off-track fartleks and tempo runs. The only speed work generally includes 4 - 6 x 100 meter strides on grass after a longer run. This phase normally lasts around two to six months, depending on the runner and his or her goals.

The next phase is the pre-comp phase. This is where the workouts are a little lower in volume, higher in intensity, generally referred to as the VO2 MAX phase. It features intervals ranging around two to ten minutes (800 meters - two miles) and more stuff done on the track but still longer intervals. Racing generally begins or has already begun in this phase but is still early in the season and mileage is generally kept high.

Personally, this phase always killed me. The increase of high-volume, high-intensity workouts killed me. This phase normally spans one to two months and in my opinion, lasts one to two months too long. Some runners do very well in races off of this type of work though, but not this *harrier*. In any case, this phase is not for me.

> Harrier: I never actually knew what a harrier was until I looked it up and discovered several definitions. Among them are: A bird of prey; a hawk, which flies low over meadows and marshes to hunt small mammals or birds; a runner, specifically, a cross country runner; a dog; a vertical take-off and landing fighter jet. I like the hawk and jet definitions the best.
> "Running… is the closest man will ever get to flying."
> ~ Joseph VanderStel

Then we have my personal favorite phase, the sharpening/racing period. This phase is generally low in volume, high in intensity, 30 second to 2-minute intervals (200 - 800 meter), normally ran on the track at race pace or faster. It generally takes place toward the end of the season, near championship races, so mileage is cut down, tempos and fartleks are shorter in time increments, fast-base runs are cut down or taken out entirely. Generally lactate tolerance and speed-endurance work, Fast Twitch Type II and fast Twitch Type IIB Muscle fibers (speed and speed endurance) are worked on in this phase.

If a runner is kept in this phase too long, burnout will soon ensue, which is probably why so many coaches seem to fear it. Runners will burnout the fastest in this phase because of the rapid adaptations the body makes. Also, the excess waste produced by the muscles from the speed work can linger and wreak havoc on the body. The key is to know is that this phase is the best and most effective, but if you do not know how to optimize it, you can go backwards, down hill, in a Red Ryder wagon off of a cliff. This is no reason to avoid or be scared of the sharpening and speed phase, but it is a major reason why research is essential; learn as much as you can about it. And sometimes, like me, one must use good old-fashioned trial and error, because, if you want to increase your success rate, you have to increase your failure rate. This phase generally lasts two to six weeks. Then, you start over again at phase 1, and that is a typical runner's cycle.

I think this last phase is the only reason a traditional taper works. The runner is finally doing what he needed to get faster in the last bit of their competition period. Therefore, the runner does get faster and he attributes it to a good taper. Unless the athlete is too burnt out from overtraining earlier in the season, then nothing but time off will improve speed.

The Non-Traditional Periodization Plan

Another periodization plan I've tried out on my own is the Undulated Periodization Plan. Charles Poliquin (1988) is the founder of undulated periodization. Poliquin studied professional body builders, but there is a vast array of training ideas for runners to learn about and utilize from his studies and thoughts on the subject; I did. Poliquin thought traditional periodization had loads of faults. He didn't like that any phase or cycle, like base phase in the most common plan, was not varied for at least four weeks, and in our case, sometimes up to five months!

An athlete will normally acclimate to a training stimulus in about two weeks, and as a consequence, gains diminish. I found this to be very true in my personal quest for the best training. You could remain in the base phase forever while not ever really improving much, and never feel too drained. This is probably why casual joggers spend their whole life in this phase, and someday, after competitive running, I'll be there too. And I will run for years without really getting too drained from it.

But I could wear myself out in as little as a week the VO2 Max phase and speed phase! Zatsiorsky (1995) calls this the biological law of accommodation, which states that the response of a biological object to a given stimulus decreases over time. This means, over time runners adapt to a type of training or workouts and stop improving their speed. And with the higher-intensity stuff in the later two phases, you can adapt rapidly and then go backwards just as fast. Some people say this happens over two to four weeks but I have seen it happen much faster. If you keep performing the same over time and keep working out and racing without performance increases, you will soon start to go backwards in performance and overtrain, overreach, and burnout.

Psychologists call this conditioned inhibition. It could be caused from reactive inhibition, where the body reacts to inhibit the action that causes extreme fatigue. To prevent this, runners should continually switch the focus of their training frequently, thus avoiding the boredom and mental fatigue of monotonous activity. The change also trains a different system that is not fatigued so the athlete can deter conditioned inhibition.

This type of periodizing also contributes to a continual increase in speed and intensity, resulting in an accumulation of stress, which promotes burnout. Then, the strength/base gained from the first months of training in this cycle would go down in comparison to the pre-competition, competition and championship phases. These involved higher intensities and decreasing volumes, both of which are not good for strength, rendering the first months of this periodization practically worthless.

For Non-Traditional Periodization Program, you change the focus every two to three weeks. Base includes two to three weeks; Pre-competition and VO2 work lasts two to three weeks; Taper, sharpening, and speed work should take another two to three week; then repeat the cycle.

I tried this form of periodization but could not determine when I would reach my best shape or when I would be in danger of burnout and overtraining. Ironically, I still managed to get burnt out in each phase; I didn't want to do the similar workouts each couple of weeks. By the end of the three weeks I was more than happy to be done with that phase. I decided something had to change; I did not want to cycle for two months and only have one or two peak races at random times. I figured I couldn't do the same type of workout back to back with such frequency and expect to avoid quick fatigue; I had to drastically change something within my training system, again.

My Daily Undulated Periodization Program: My Favorite

In the past, I had trained within a high-intensity speed, speed endurance, and aerobic endurance weekly regiment I really enjoyed. Still though, I felt fatigued after about a month and a half or so of the training. I had some crazy weeks: Sunday was speed endurance on the track; Monday included two tempo runs; Tuesday, I ran pure speed work at the track; Wednesday was one light active-rest run as well as one tempo/aerobic endurance run; Thursday included a speed endurance workout followed by tempo; Friday was an active-rest day; Saturday, I ran the 1200 meter time trial with pure speed afterwards.

I also did much more lifting with the legs on the track workout days. This whipped me into PHENOMENAL shape in every area very quickly. I ran a 3:41 – 1500 meter time after a month of this hard training; a five-second lifetime personal record (PR) and a 20-second season PR! I really enjoyed switching it up between aerobic endurance (slow twitch), speed endurance (fast twitch Type IIa), speed (fast twitch Type IIb) and active rest (eight to ten minute pace, simply pumps blood to the muscles you use while running recovering them very quickly).

This was a very good system; one semi-borrowed from El Guerrouj's training book, but catered to my needs. I put my specifics down on paper for the entire month I used this system. I made it from running a 4:01 – 1500 meter, feeling like the fat kid trying to catch the bus, to running a 3:41 – 1500 meter with energy to spare. I also recorded the rest of the month's training leading up to nationals that year. It was a good training system with some flaws that had to be worked out. Every training detail was recorded; I thought it could be very beneficial to see so I included it in the end of Section 1.

My daily, undulated periodization program is a system that worked very well for reasons that made complete sense to me. Aerobic endurance work and speed endurance/speed work complement each other. When you perform each as part of an integrated holistic program, you can make vast improvements on both very rapidly. The problem comes when the workouts are separated; this allows too much time in between, then both workouts suffer vastly from the absence of the other by taxing one system to frequently. I'm not sure if there is any research about this scenario, but it just makes sense to me based on personal experience in my own training, as well as considering how some of the fastest runners put their workouts together.

Logically, this makes sense to me on a basic common training sense level. Runners and coaches alike will agree that slower aerobic distance work reduces a runner's speed from ignoring the anaerobic fast twitch muscles, and instead, builds his or her slow twitch muscles predominantly. Respectively, most coaches and runners know that speed work hurts endurance and slow twitch muscle fibers by focusing on fast twitch muscle fibers. So when paired together, they can grow together; keep them separated and previous gains will diminish. This separation is an all too common mistake in a conventional running program. For me, since I was building up every area very aggressively simultaneously, I improved in every area of my running at the same time.

The only problem that remained was fatigue. I was still mentally and physically tired throughout the season. I think this again can be attributed to adapting quickly to training stimulus, however, I did stay fit much longer than normal. I lasted about two months the first time I tried it, racing pretty well and having pretty good workouts.

When I tried it the following year, I lasted from late March/early April into late July. I ran a 3:41 – 1500 meter a couple times, and a 1:47 – 800 meter several times through those four months. My speed increased quickly, but then plateaued for a long time. Physically, it was a toss-up. Sometimes I felt crappy and tight for some workouts but did great, and other moments, I felt fully rested and non-achy and then I'd run with lead shoes! I didn't get it. But I still wanted to remain in this type of training. I simply had to figure out how to avoid hitting a plateau and overtraining, while still improving my speed throughout the season and be able to knowledgably peak for races throughout the year. (Most coaches and athletes will agree, peaking is one of the hardest things to do.)

The Eureka Moment

I began coaching at Los Gatos High School with the great Karl Keska and he told me that he liked to take a break in training for a whole week every four to six weeks of hard training. I thought that was brilliant and as it turned out, this was the missing link in my training program. I had been taking a day or two off with just active rest or slow base days but this was not long enough to get away from the mental stresses of hard training and racing because I was still worrying about the next time I was going to hammer a tempo run, or light up the track with a hard workout or a big race at the end of those couple days off.

Four to seven days off, however, provides ample time to fully recover from a high-intensity training system like this where every system is pushed to the limits every day. I changed the plan and worked through two or three weeks maximum of high-intensity training with a long break at the end. Happily, I felt pretty stinking good at the end of this break and was excited to get back to the track. But man, when I re-started the hard workouts was I flat! My times sucked in workouts and then slowly improved after a few. This led to my non-conventional taper for races and plateau buster for continued gains throughout the season.

The Completely Shererious Taper

I remembered how good I felt for some workouts in the middle of my previous training and how flat I felt after I took a couple of light days before a race. This coincided with how I felt after I took some time off to recover after this cycle. I decided to take a four-day taper the week before a race, and then train my butt off the week of the race. I did a high-intensity, long-rest speed workout two days before the meet to help my legs feel snappy and get used to a quicker than race pace.

This worked amazingly well. I felt pretty good and springy for the Husky Invitational, the first race where I tried out this taper. During the race, the sub 60 second per lap pace felt very slow, because of the 10 x 200 meter at 27 – 24 seconds, 48 hours prior to race time. Sitting comfortably in the lead pack, I took off and ran a very fast last 500 meters to run a 3:56.0 mile; this was early a six-second lifetime PB, and the fastest time in the world that year, as well as the fastest time run indoor by an American that year or the previous year. I had not gotten any faster in the mile since 2004, four years ago, and I had just earned the fourth fastest first sub-four minute mile time in history for an American.

I continued to do this throughout the season and experienced some bad racing strategies and misfortune in the races, but I was still fit; possibly the best information and result that I could ask for in the quest to perfect my training.

The training system I currently use is very similar to the extremely detailed one I include at the end of this Section. The things I tweaked to fine tune include: limiting myself to two track workouts a week and an additional weekly hill workout. I'll put a race in there too if I can find one and it works well with my schedule. To prepare for races, I run repeat 200 meters fast two days prior, with as much rest as I want in between intervals. Of course, I add a longer down time periodically throughout the season to destroy mental and physical fatigue.

Rodger Banister (1975) had a two factor mathematical theory on human performance: Performance = Fitness - Fatigue. This is a good theory, but I think it's missing something. Banister's model works for the traditional taper of progressively cutting down volume and frequency while slightly increasing intensity. This will keep fitness levels and reduce fatigue possibly, but the body will be adapting to less and less strenuous workouts. This could lead to a loss of readiness in the athlete.

Tim Noakes talked about a central governor in his book, *Lore of Running: 4th Edition*, that shuts down the heart and lungs before any muscle or organ damage could be done from pushing it too hard. This is based on what the body knows it can handle and other unknown factors. This fits his model in that the brain would be adapting to less and less stress making the extreme stresses of a race more of a shock to the system, which in turn would make the governor shut the body down before it actually could. Because of this, I would like to add the readiness factor to Banister's model. Performance = Fitness - Fatigue + Readiness. This makes my taper the best because it gives you a rest to reduce fatigue, while increasing fitness and readiness leading up to the race which equals a better performance. Boo-ya.

This taper is a good taper. I find that during the season a mid-distance runner should generally keep the same pace for the season and the same volume. The little four to five day breaks/tapers should keep the runner fresh for the whole season to not burn out. As the season moves along, the athlete should feel more and more refreshed as his or her body adapts to the same pace and workouts.

Racing should also be considered one of the best workouts for the athlete. Making sure they do not go too fast and start racing workouts is a difficult and essential component. Often, as athletes get fitter and the workouts get easier, they will want to go faster. This could burn an athlete out in a hurry. I prefer to stay between a mile pace and a little faster than an 800 meter race pace, but not too much faster. I have found that going at a 400 meter pace or faster for a mid-distance runner can really hurt race performance if held too long. I would suggest only running this pace occasionally.

Again, be careful; as athletes adapt to the race pace and goal race pace training, the tendency is to go too hard and too long in workouts. Even training by myself, I have made an error in this area and ruined the last bit of my season because of it. At the end of the season, you should be hitting the times you were hitting at the start, but it should be easier with less residual fatigue. Unlike the normal model of training where you do long stuff to build endurance and then destroy that period with pure speed at the end of the year, you keep everything getting stronger and you should be feeling better. The race times should be getting faster, but practice times should only improve a little bit, if at all.

The main workouts to focus on are speed endurance and speed workouts that range from mile race pace to slightly faster than 800 race pace. I have a couple workouts that seem to work very well for me and make it easy to get in 2000 to 4000 meters of race pace or faster per workout. I've learned to not change the volume or pace of these workouts too much at the end of the season. I have included all of my workouts in the next section. I don't have too many, but I really don't think you need a bunch of different workouts to "keep it fresh" or "develop the whole athlete;" you just need a couple of the right ones.

1. Poliquin, C. "Five steps to increasing the effectiveness of your strength training program." NSCA J. 10:34–39. 1988.
2. Zatsiorsky, Vladimir. "Science And Practice Of Strength Training." Human Kinetics. 1995
3. Banister, E. W., Calvert, T. W., Savage, M. V. (1975) "A systems model of training for athletic performance." J. Sports. Med. 7, p.57-61.

Lane 3

Workouts:
Intervals, Tempos, Fartleks, and Long Runs, Oh My!

There are a million different workouts for a million different things. It's like a sandwich, with many different ways to make each part of the sandwich and some taste similar and others, some vastly different. For me, there are four categories of running workouts: aerobic endurance (bread), speed endurance (peanut butter), speed (jelly) and active rest (banana). These four merge together to make the best sandwich ever, a peanut butter and jelly with a baseball bat. You can catch the theme song for this sandwich online with the popular dancing banana. But for these different categories of training, I will explain what each of them and how they will help you improve so you can build a better program for yourself.

Aerobic Endurance (AE)

Aerobic endurance primarily addresses your slow twitch Type I muscle fibers, your base. I'm not going to go into great scientific detail about all the little things you work on at a cellular level; that stuff is good to know and I have researched it so I'll try to present a good top-level picture for you. This work increases endurance and allows you to do more speed endurance and gain speed on the track.

I can see where some people look at a glutton for speed like my-self and think that I will say this is the least important. Well, some people are wrong; this is very important work. I do agree with coaches who feel that the more base you can do, the more speed you can do later. I also agree this kind of work allows you to do more of the performance-enhancing, speedy track work, which is why this type of training should be done quite often during intense track training. During a random week (5/14 - 5/20) from my hard training program, I did six AE workouts, six recovery runs and on-ly three speedy track workouts. The emphasis, ratio wise, was on AE and recovery runs, but that work allowed me to log nearly 10,000 meters of mile race pace or faster on the track that week.

My rule of thumb for aerobic endurance workouts is to never run this pace on the track. Aerobic endurance work is slower than mile and 800 race pace, and I do not want to get used to going slow on the track. This means that any workout with intervals over 600 meters are run off of the track. My advice for you is to never get used to running anything slower than goal race pace or faster on the track. I believe running slower on the track can lead to condi-tioned and reactive inhibition for races.

If you're training your body to get extremely fatigued doing slower paces on the track, how do you think it will react when you pick up the pace in a race? Odds are your alarm reaction to the in-creased intensity will shut down your bodies function far before it is near being super fatigued. This feels like somebody's giving you a big hug while trying to breath; legs tie up and can't turn over, the heart rate drops, the entire body tenses up, and then shortly after the race you feel fine. I'm sure all runners have experienced this before, and no, it's not because "you didn't want it enough," or "you didn't compete!" It is because your training was not optimal for you and/or your race.

The workouts for this vary quite a bit. My two favorites are the cut-down/tempo and fartlek. Fartlek is Swedish for speed play and is a type of continuous conditioning. For a tempo/cutdown, I'll run 15 – 30 minutes from 4:50 – 5:45 pace, depending on how I feel that day.

I don't always time these either though, but I have out of pure curiosity. I think it's better to let your body decide how fast it wants to run, as opposed to using a watch and a preconceived notion. With the latter, when you're not going as fast as you previously ran (this will happen), you might be tempted to push it harder than your body on needs to that particular day to order to feel better about yourself during the run. Doing this could hinder your interval workouts the next day. I call them Tempo runs sometimes, but I always build into it to see how I feel so it's basically always a cut-down in all honesty. I like cut-down runs un-timed so I can build into the workout without pressure and then if I feel better I can pick it up. If I don't, I maintain or slow down if I'm really fried.

My weekly fartlek generally entails going up a mountain, running the hard parts up the hill and jogging the easy parts down the hill. I like to run four or five sets of the following, in minute increments: 1 minute on, 1 minute off; 2 on, 1 off; 1 on, 1 off; 3 on, 1 off. This is one of my favorite workouts for aerobic endurance and I'll tell you why.

On average, runners will do this work on the track repeating a mile, or 1200, 1000, or 800 meters many times. This is pretty hard on the body; I know this from personal experience. Because of the length of the interval, it's very hard to actually increase intensity on the track or even maintain it. When a runner knows the distance of the repeat and how fast he or she should run it, a runner will typically push it a bit harder than his or her body can handle to hit the times he or she thinks ought to be hit. Running off the track and up hill, a runner will go much slower than race pace, but they really have no idea what pace they're going. They just push it for that amount of time how hard their body wants to push.

For me, some intervals are a lot slower than others, but I am always breathing hard and going up fast, getting in a good aerobic workout. If runners become slaves to hitting certain times for certain distances in this type of workout, they will not be able to listen to their body as much. I do time my speed workouts on the track, but they are not as long, and not potentially draining, mentally, so I'm not too worried. But perhaps it would be a good idea to skip on timing my speedy track intervals as well. I'll talk to my coach about it.

Along with this workout, sometimes I just run up a mountain for two minutes, then jog back down and repeat the route. This work is basically slower than race pace work; generally I run it at a 4:30 to 6:30 minute mile pace, but I rarely time it. Again, I wouldn't recommend timing and taking the pace too seriously; time isn't important for this workout. The effort is important, not the pace. Keep tempos comfortable and quick; you should make fartleks a little more challenging so really push it. My fartleks will last around an hour, but since the process broken up with very easy jogging, it's not as strenuous on the body as a continuous AE run. Unlike a continuous run, fartleks include high-intensity and recovery portions so the body has recovery time from the stimulus,

This is also where the long run comes in. I don't do them nor recommend them. I think the long run should be abolished for runners who race five miles or less. For reasons I've stated earlier, it's just worse on your body to train it to run long and slow. My high school coach once said: "long slow running makes long slow runners," and I completely agree. While this may be a good way to keep the weight off, you put so much cortisol into your system that you're in a catabolic state for a while afterwards burning away your fat and muscle. This can be different for everybody though but this could explain why long-distance runners look like those starving kids in charity commercials. On the other end of the spectrum, muscle-bound sprinters rarely reach that catabolic state, and mid-distance runners are typically, well, in the middle. More research needs to be done on this as well. Curiosity demands an answer.

Speed Endurance

In this phase, you are primarily working on your fast twitch Type IIa muscle fibers. These are your speed endurance muscle fibers; they allow you to hold your speed for longer duration. They are the middle muscles for the mid-distance runner. Type I last a long time, but don't produce enough power; Type IIb produce the most power but fatigue very quickly; and Type IIa are just right.

If you race the 800 meters and up, Type IIa fibers are essential. You will work on your fast twitch Type IIb and your slow twitch Type I muscle fibers as well but just not as much. Fast twitch Type IIa fibers are the hardest to train and grow; in my opinion they are the most important muscle type and that is what speed endurance workouts are for.

In speed endurance workouts, you're also working on pacing and adapting your body to the pace you want to run for your race. It's important to let your body know it can handle the pace. There are many ways to do this type of workout: if you take more rests, you work more on speed; if you take shorter rests, you work on more endurance. I like to keep it equal or longer rest vs. interval time. I like this type of workout at the start of the week and then run quicker, shorter, and less distance (speed) at the end of the week. I do this mainly because races are typically at the end of a week and I want my speed work closest to the race. That makes the quick pace of races seem less intense if the last time you were on the track you went faster than race pace. After this workout, it's good to do a very slow recovery run, and possibly another one that night too.

There are not too many workouts for this type of work in my opinion. I only vary two different workouts for this work. I think a good workout to do before you start racing is Bannister's 10 x 400 meter workout around 60 second pace. He took two minutes in between intervals, while El Guerrouj only took 30 seconds and ran around 52-53 second pace they say... Sick! I prefer to go in the middle and take one minute keeping it a 60 second pace. This workout is ridiculously hard, and should not be done too often. I really only do this workout a few times in preseason. I pretty much let my races equal this workout in a season. If you do it in the middle of a season I think it might take too much out of you.

My favorite workout for speed endurance, which I do once a week, is one given to me by a local high school coach named Willie Harmatz; it consists of 200 and 300 meter runs. This one I run 300 meter – 200 meter x 6, starting at race pace or slower and moving to slightly faster than race pace. I begin each interval at the same spot on the track and have different jogging rests for recovery. The faster the jog, the more Aerobic Endurnace benefits.

Those are the two workouts I run, often varying them slightly, depending on how I feel and if I want to switch it up a little. If you're really hurting in the middle of this workout, it's better to take a longer break, do it later in the day, or stop instead of pushing through. It will come around with time, but remember, the muscle fibers we are targeting here are slow to develop so keep at it.

This workout is key, so I will try to help you with the pacing for it. At the beginning of the season, I have to really push it to hit the times, and as the season moves along, it gets easier. I try to get to a place where I can start around 43 seconds for the 300 meter and 28 seconds for the 200 meter, which is slightly faster than 1500 meter race pace, and then finish around 41 seconds for the 300 meter and 27 seconds for the 200 meter on the last couple intervals. That's about 800-meter race pace for me. This workout does not take too much away from the athlete and still gives him or her 3000 meters of faster than mile race pace work. B. E. A. Utiful! I like to add five times one hundred meters at the start too. This helps with warm up and adds another 500 meters of pace work for a grand total of 3,500 meters of race pace or faster. The best thing is that it doesn't take too much out of you if you do it right. Too fast and you're in a hurt locker without a key.

Speed: I Feel a Need

My old roommate Nick Willis (Silver medalist in the 1500 meters at the Beijing Olympic Games) once called me a glutton for speed, and I would agree with his analysis of the situation. I love cranking it on the track. I love watching things rapidly go by me and turning my legs over quickly; I just want to go fast.

Speed endurance training works primarily on your fast twitch type IIa and IIb muscle fibers, but also works slow twitch and is found to be better for the heart than long aerobic work! Some would say this type of training works on your VO2 Max and AE far better than moderate-intensity continuous running. Based on common sense alone, I would agree but there are also many studies that support that theory. If you're making your body adapt to higher intensities, going longer at lower intensities will feel and be easier. Likewise, if a boxer is accustomed to being punched in the face frequently, getting slapped in the face wouldn't be too bad. The boxer would probably handle multiple slaps, as opposed to well-practiced slap fighter, if there was such a thing, whose world be rocked by a solid hard punch, a total shock to the system.

This is explanation for why I think speed endurance is the most important work you can do. Obviously, a laboratory study needs to be done on punch vs. slap training.

High-intensity training, being the most beneficial to performance because of quick adaptations, can also be the most dangerous if you do not know how to wield its awesome power. Like I said, most coaches veer away from this work because it's very easy to over tax your system and burnout fast on this work. I will explain how to avoid burnout and still reap the benefits of speed work all year long in a moment.

There are plenty of different workouts I do for this, but typically I only do 100 and 200 meter distances; rest is user preference. Quality is a little more important here than having a set recovery time. I read it takes approximately four minutes to completely replenish the adenosine tripnosphate (ATP) and creatine stores in your muscles so you can keep performance up without destroying all your glycogen stores, but I still think it really should be based on how you feel.

I used to take my heart rate and would wait until it was around 115 beats per minute before I started the next interval. Now I just wait until I feel ready to go as fast or faster for the next interval. But starting off with the heart-rate idea did provide valuable internal feedback on how I felt. My all-time favorite speed workout is

10 x 200 meters. I like to keep it around 800-meter race pace; I start out a little slower, and end a little faster. I really feel this is all you need to get in a great speed workout.

I know various coaches and athletes swear by 300 meters, 400 meters and 600 meters done at the 800 meter race pace or faster, but I think this hurts performance by making your body VERY fatigued at that pace. Repeating 200-meter runs at the 800-meter goal pace won't tire out good athletes. They could probably do even more total volume even faster doing 200 meters at this pace than the longer intervals.

A popular workout that I think is muy malo is a set of four x 400 meter in around 50 – 53 seconds. A workout like this can be very taxing and might put you in the hole for a while, possibly leading to burnout soon thereafter; from only 1600 meters total! My beautiful workout is 2000 meters at 49 – 52 second pace work and I can do it two days before a race without harming my performance at all since it doesn't leave very much residual fatigue. Which one sounds better on paper and based off of common sense?

I don't even need to get technical and talk about the physiological benefits of my workout over the first one, but I will because I'm a bit of a nerd. In my run, going that pace for less than 30 seconds uses mainly ATP and creatine as a fuel source, which means you use less glycogen. Because of the breaks, you also don't build up too many dangerous hydrogen radicals in your blood. The right muscles for speed endurance are still being worked because it's over 12 second intervals and the amount of work done at that speed plays a factor as well. Additionally, the heart is trained to stay high throughout the interval instead of shutting down in the middle when the body perceives it is in danger.

In the first workout, running 400 meters at 800 meter race pace or faster can completely diminish an athlete's glycogen stores very quickly. If glycogen stores are gone, the body will shut down and take a long time to recover from the depletion; it could take weeks or even months. The mental agony of feeling the body shut down at that pace could result in an additional set back as well. So in my self-proclaimed expert opinion, this is a dangerous workout with minimal return; a bad investment.

Coe and El Guerrouj had a similar workout with 300 meters instead of 200 meters. El G did them in 35 to 36 seconds and didn't say how long he took to rest. I assume it was similar to mine, different every time. My fastest ever is a 37 seconds; sad. But even going that fast for a 300 meter in a workout seems to hang on me a while after the workout. This makes me all the more scared to even try a 400-meter at that pace in a workout. Coe and El G seemed to do well with it so the training may be a good alternative for some people; I just know it's not for me.

Another workout I run is a series of 100-meter straights. This is where you jog around the track in eighth lane and sprint the 100-meter straights. I normally do 8 – 12 total straights as a very easy track workout on my taper week, or sometimes only five straights as a warm up to add a little more volume to my total speed on the track. Some times a use them to build all out pure speed, but it tears up your hamstrings and quads something awful, so if you do it, be careful! They don't use much glycogen, but they can leave you sore for a good long time afterwards.

Active Rest

This running really doesn't work on any of the different muscle fibers specifically, but it does recover all of them. Active rest is dirt-slow running, around an 8 – 10 minute mile pace. All this running does is pump blood to the muscles without depleting glycogen stores. This greatly speeds recovery! It is very effective to do this type of running in between harder runs that took a lot out of you. This pace is also good for a pre-race shake-out or warm-up run; it also serves well after a hard workout, or if you're just feeling awful. I heard that Kenyans run for two hours at this pace on their off days and recover faster than if they'd just took a day off completely. You won't catch me running this pace over 30 minutes, but I do agree that it's a great way to recover faster. While going on these runs I have been passed by many older, heavier, and slower joggers and you just have to suck up your pride, know what you're trying to accomplish with this type of run and do it.

I have also read that while going on these slow runs, you are going slowly enough to burn fat as energy and replenish your glycogen stores faster than if you did nothing. I have also read that there is no such thing as a fat-burning zone and you only burn fat at complete rest. But I tend to agree with the first theory; along with pumping blood, vitamins, nutrients, oxygen, and glycogen to the tired muscles, this slow pace teaches your body to use fat as an energy source. It also clears the free radicals that might have collected from the intense training and racing.

All in all, this pace is a must for the serious runner for a number of reasons. I have been made fun of plenty of times for running at this pace, but that doesn't really matter when you know the science behind it. People make fun of what they don't understand, and sometimes make fun of what they do understand. But do it regardless to recover.

Implementation: Putting it all Together

I guess the biggest question now might be: "How do I make this system work for me/my athletes?" Good question. I'm glad you asked! As you know, every runner is different and will like different parts of their training. Some love lighting it up on the track, others could do hard base runs all week long and be happy. This training can work for both types of runners. The holistic approach allows them to work on strengths and have those build their weaknesses. I used to get destroyed running base runs with the Michigan State team when the distance guys would start to push it. By doing this program I am able to do six runs per week at a quicker pace than I was able to go with them. I only ran maybe two or three hard base runs with the guys at MSU per week and they would wipe me out.

Since you work on every part at once, the road warriors can have a field day on the roads and hammer on the AE runs while the speedy runners can blow out some faster long rest intervals on the track. The speedy guys will most likely enjoy the track work more and might rock the distance guys on it a little bit. You have to be careful mixing the groups though; sometimes distance guys love to push recovery runs or cut downs to hard and this will greatly hurt the speed athlete.

If it's a timed rest, then let them do whatever to prepare for the next interval. The speedy guys can ruin a distance guy by dropping them on the shorter fast stuff. Make sure the distance guys don't get carried away with trying to match the speedy guys. They have to be careful on the AE runs as well though. If a runner red lines on this run, it will tire him out too much, distance or speed runner. Sometimes doing these runs with other teammates isn't always a good idea. One guy in the group will always feel great and the other runners might not want or be able to go as fast as the best feeling guy that day. This could lead to burnout in even your fastest runner when he feels like he has to go with a guy that might not race as fast, but feels good that day. Nobody really ever feels great everyday for a host of reasons, but pushing it on the days you feel awful will not help you.

This is also where the watch (especially GPS watches) can get you in trouble. If you have a set pace you think you should run because previous training dictates or a book said so, then you won't listen to your body. This will allow the cortisol to build up faster and burn you out more quickly. My base runs can often be as fast a 4:45 per mile for two or three miles when I'm really feeling great. If I tried to hit that every time, I'd be learning to walk on my hands by now. Some days I go as slow as 6:45 mile pace when I'm feeling bad and call it an AE run. If I vary two minutes per mile for these cut-down/tempo runs imagine how a team of runners who will all feel differently each day could potentially burn each other out with these runs.

The only run that you can put everyone together and not worry too much is the recovery run (RR). This dirt-slow running is used to recover from both of these high-intensity aerobic and anaerobic runs. It will be beneficial for every type of runner. The only thing to worry about is the guys who don't pay attention up front and start to drop the pace a bit. Make sure they know that the only goal is recovery, and if you go slightly too fast, you've failed. Tell the guys in the back to be vocal to the one-steppers up front (one stepper = a runner that cannot let another person run next to them or in front of them and must be one step ahead at all times).

In my hard weeks, I would do about six of these runs. It's my opinion that a serious runner should do two runs a day and an AE or RR should always be one of them. The body will let the runner know which run it should do that day but the runner needs to learn how to listen. This is where self-discipline or/and amazing coaching comes into play. Most serious runners will have the passion to run themselves into the ground. The trick is learning to listen to your body to push it the hardest it can take without going over the edge.

Here is a very basic 26-day training system:

Day 1
AM - *Speed Endurance* + Lower body weights.
PM - Recovery Run

Day 2
AM - Recovery Run
Mid-day - Aerobic Endurance + Upper body weights
PM - Recovery Run

Day 3
AM - Aerobic Endurance
PM - Aerobic Endurance

Day 4
AM - *Speed* + Lower body weights
PM - Aerobic Endurance

Day 5
AM - Recovery Run
PM - Aerobic Endurance + Upper body weights

Day 6
AM - Aerobic Endurance

PM - Recovery Run

Day 7
AM - *Hill Fartlek* + Lower body weights
PM - Aerobic Endurance

Day 8
AM - Aerobic Endurance + Upper body workout
PM - Recovery Run

Day 9
AM - *Speed Endurance* + Lower body workout
PM - Recovery run

Day 10
AM - Aerobic Endurance
PM - Aerobic Endurance + Upper body workout
Evening - Recovery Run

Day 11
AM - *Speed* + Lower body weights
PM - Aerobic Endurance

Day 12
AM - Recovery Run
Mid - Day Recovery Run
PM - Aerobic Endurance + Upper body weights

Day 13
AM - Hill Fartlek + Lower body weights
PM - Recovery Run

Day 14
AM - Aerobic Endurance
PM - Aerobic Endurance + Upper body weights

Day 15
AM - *Speed Endurance* + Lower body workout
PM - Recovery Run

Day 16
AM - Recovery Run
PM - Recovery Run

Day 17
AM - Recovery Run
PM - Recovery Run

Day 18
AM - Recovery Run + 8 x 100 meter strides
PM - Recovery Run

Day 19
AM - Recovery Run
PM - Recovery Run

Day 20
AM - *Hill Fartlek* + Lower body weights
PM - Recovery Run

Day 21
AM - Aerobic Endurance + Upper body weights
PM - Recovery Run

Day 22
AM - *Speed Endurance* + Lower body weights
PM - Recovery Run

Day 23
AM - Aerobic Endurance
PM - Aerobic Endurance

Day 24
AM - *Speed*
PM - Recovery Run

Day 25
AM - Recovery Run
Mid Day - Recovery Run
PM - Recovery Run

Day 26
AM - *Race Day*
PM - Recovery Run

This is like a recipe; sometimes you have to give it a personal touch to make it the best recipe for you. Some AE run will turn into RR workouts, and some speed workouts will turn into RR workouts. I would recommend always going less intense when changing the plan; too much intensity, even when you're feeling great, is a recipe for burnout.

Some runners may require more AE runs because they thrive off of longer lower-intensity runs. Others may need more all-out pure speed work and can build up from there. Personally, I have found that right down the middle is the best for me. I like to do Speed Endurance workouts the most. Even at the end of a season, I'll try to avoid the high amounts of speed that most runners do. I just keep doing the same paces and volumes; my body adapts to it better. For instance, I found if I go faster than 25 for a 200 meter, it hurts my performance. And if I go faster than 40 for a 300 meter, it doesn't really help me at all. But doing several reps at 26 – 28 seconds for a 200 meter and 41 – 43 seconds for a 300 meter suits me perfectly.

Lane 4

Got Gym?
Weight Training for Runners

This is probably going to be the longest chapter and possibly the most in-depth. I am a gym rat. I really enjoy getting in the weight room and cranking out a great workout as fast and as intense as I can. I feel good after it, I feel good during it, and I even enjoy thinking about the next time I'm going to get in there and work on something different. I have a Masters in Kinesiology (the study of human movement); am a NASM (National Association of Sports Medicine) Certified Personal Trainer; and most importantly, I thoroughly enjoy reading the latest research articles online, talking with experienced trainers and lifters, watching other people in the weight room, and training others. And being a world-class runner, I think I have the most to offer fellow runners in this area.

At the gym, there are many things runners can do to increase and improve strength, stability, mind-body connection, power, VO2 MAX, bone strength, tendon/ligament durability, muscle recruitment, and even psychological state. The weight room will not automatically make you a better runner; nothing can substitute the time you put into a sport-specific action, a.k.a, running. But it will help you stay injury free, and increase overall fitness, namely all the things I just listed above.

Many coaches will tell their runners something like "lifting will only make you gain weight and get slow," or "you don't need to lift, only running can make you faster." In my opinion, those coaches are basically saying: "I don't really know what I'm doing in the weight room, and I don't want to research it to see what it's all about. Plus, I knew some great runners who never touched the weights." And in all honesty, that's a valid response; if you don't know what you're doing, it's probably not good to just go out there and do something you think might work. You can get hurt if you do not know what you're doing in the weight room. Also, there are in fact great runners who never touch the weight room.

However, I strongly believe every runner could benefit from a weight routine catered to what they like and want to develop. More importantly, the weight room is your best doctor for recovering from injuries, as well as avoiding repeat injuries. In my opinion, weight training helps injuries more than icing, myofascial release, deep-tissue massage, ultra-sound, cortisone shots, and surgery (unless unavoidable but kiss your running career goodbye). It's the same with stretching or really all the other forms of recovery that don't incorporate your body adapting to stimulus to make it stronger and help it build up the muscles, tendons, and ligaments around the affected area.

If you make your body dependent on outside stimulus to perform, it will adapt to that and you will be weaker in the long run, even if it helps at the start. Your body is an amazing thing, and it can adapt to amazing things. If you give your body a more challenging stimulus, like lifting, it will adapt to that and become stronger. If you make it easier than normal for your body, it will adapt to that and become weaker. Go for the harder permanent fix instead of the quick fix that keeps you injured for the long run. Pun intended.

Upper Body

I will first start with the upper body since there's not as much as the lower body to write about it. Contrary to popular running belief, lifting with your upper body can be very beneficial to runners. It is actually the only way to work out the thoracic cavity in your chest, which in turn can increase your VO2 max. Just lifting with your lower body will not do this. And lifting incorrectly with your upper body will not do this. It's good to lift with compound upper body movement with no recovery between different workouts with as many sets and reps as you can do.

Navy Seal Tier II Workout

This is pretty much the only workout I do for upper body, or variations of this workout. It's simply four upper-body workouts done as fast as possible. Do 30 push ups, 35 full sit ups, 20 dips, and 10 pull ups as fast as you can and repeat six times. I generally do this in around 20 minutes or less. All these movements use just about all your upper body, but make sure you contract your abs and back muscles during all the movements. Doing single muscle exercises like bicep curls, triceps extensions, shrugs, and other such single muscle exercises can get you larger and will not workout your thoracic cavity as well. I do variations of this workout; I generally try to get more reps in than sets. I currently do 50 push ups, 20 dips, 30 pull ups and 50 sit ups, and do this 3 or 4 times as fast as I can. I do not have huge arms, but I do have a fit upper body, and my breathing has come a long way because of it. I have sports induced asthma, but since I've been doing this workout, I have had much less problems breathing, except for one time at the Olympic trials. But in that case, there were other contributing factors, which I'll go over later.

Push-ups: Hands wide enough to get a perfect 90-degree angle in your elbow when down all the way. You can go a little further if you want, but speed and reps are more important than form. Keep back and abs contracted, butt down, and blow air out hard on the way up. Go as fast as possible. Try to keep your face as relaxed as possible.

Sit-ups: Keep you lower back flexed and pulled in. Abs contracted; your focus on these muscles the whole time. The more you focus on your abs, the more you will work them and be able to utilize them while running. Reach your shoulder blades back and keep your lower back off of the ground. This will work out your whole core a bit more than just rolling up. Blow air out of lungs and contract your abs to do so on the way up. Stay relaxed.

Dips: Use dip handles or a bench if you can't find one. Keep abs and back flexed. Try to get a 90-degree angle in your elbow on the way down, and push yourself right back up. Blow air out on the way up and relax. You can do behind the back dips on a chair or bench if you do not have dips handles or it's too hard for you.

Pull-ups: Wide grip palms facing away from you for pull-ups, and narrow grip palms facing you for chin-ups. Both are good and you should switch between the two periodically during the workout. Get down to about 90 degrees or more and pull yourself up to where your hands are around face level. Speed and reps are more important than form, but don't swing around. Keep abs contracted to stop from swinging around. Blow air out on the way up and relax your face.

Obliques:

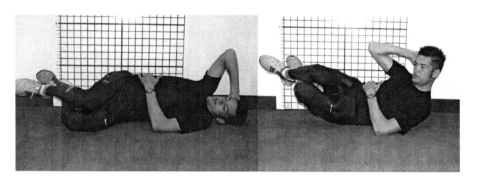

After I do all of the push-ups, sit-ups, dips, and pull-ups, I like to work on my oblique muscles. To do this, just lie on your side. Use your elbow that's on the ground to balance and put your hand in front of you. Next, get your body as high as you can sideways by pushing your hips off the ground. The higher you get the harder it is. Cross your legs and pull them up with your upper body. Put the hand that's up on your head and try to push your elbow into your hip. I'll do this 50-75 times each side. Focus on flexing your side muscles the entire time. Make 'em burn.

Lower Body

This is obviously the more important of the two parts for running and there's much more that goes into putting together a proper routine for your lower body to make it perform to its optimum and stay injury free.

Some things enter the equation that one should consider like periodization: determining which muscles to workout first, which muscles to workout last, and which exercises to perform at the right times. Also, form is much more important for your lower body exercises than your upper body. If you perform a squat, lunge, leg press, step-up, or any other loaded bent-knee exercise, you can damage the knee joint if the exercise is not done correctly. If you do too many power exercises in a week or month's time, you can damage all your joints, particularly your Achilles tendon. If you do not have the strength and ligament/tendon built up prior to power exercises, you are putting yourself at risk for extreme muscle/tendon/ligament pulls, tears, even snaps. For this reason, periodization is critical when starting out a weight routine. After your body adapts to all the types of training you can do an undulated periodization plan, which mixes it up between the 3 phases throughout the week.

Phase I: Stability, Coordination, and Mind-Body Connection

Phase One will work on your coordination by putting you in controlled unstable movements, causing you to utilize stability muscles to catch yourself. This will strengthen your tendons and ligaments before you add more weight and stress on them through muscle endurance and power phases. By utilizing all the different muscles to stabilize yourself, you increase your mind-body connection by training your brain to utilize muscles that it normally does not use. This will improve your running by helping you acquire more muscles for your stride you otherwise would not use. It will also help you be a more coordinated, symmetrical runner by getting rid of muscle imbalances. It is important to start in this phase for about two to four weeks until you're balanced and coordinated before you move on to strength and power routines.

Phase II: Muscle Endurance

In Phase Two, you are working on your muscle strength and endurance together. This is where you add weight and do many sets and reps. Begin with low weight and move up. Keep reps and sets high at all times. I generally do 3-6 sets with 20 reps in each set for the larger muscles, and then 1-2 sets for the smaller muscle groups. The focus is more on the larger muscle groups in this phase; you worked on the smaller ones more in the stability phase. However, never ever leave them out of this phase; it is very important that you work on them in this phase as well, especially if you had or have problems with a certain muscle group.

Some examples of problems include: Achilles tendinitis, shin splints, plantar fasciitis issues, or gastrocnemius issues. If you have had problems with any of these, take these exercises very seriously, and strengthen the area or it will become a chronic and possibly permanent injury. The first time you lift with the area, it will be sore! I had one athlete stop because he said it hurt it worse, and of course, it's going to hurt if you've never strengthen the area before. You have to break down the muscles to build them back stronger.

Anytime you start a strength routine (or power exercises, or running, or anything else physical that your body isn't used to), your body will be sore, potentially very sore for one to four days afterwards. You will adapt and this will go away with time. Don't quit and don't sit around and chat or wait for somebody else to get done with an exercise before doing the next set or rep of an opposing or different muscle group. Go through it with perfect form, but still as fast as possible. Research has shown that HGH and T are released in greater amounts when exercises are done on different muscle groups with no rest in between. This will not make you bigger, but will help you adapt faster and gain more from the workout. It also gives you a better cardiovascular workout as well. You really don't ever want to lift too much over 30-45 minutes, so if you're in there for an hour you might be chatting too much or sitting around letting yourself recover. Be on point. Wear head phones if people keep talking to you; they won't talk to you if you're wearing headphones. Also, avoid extended eye contact; just give a quick wave and get back to work. This is a polite way of saying, I acknowledge your presence, and I will talk with you in a bit, but right now I have to get this done. Be intense!

Phase III: Power

This phase is the most sport-specific and can give you the most gains as a runner. With more power you can have fewer strides per mile, which in turn makes you a more efficient and faster runner. Power = Strength x Speed. Without a proper strength base, you will not have a good power output. If you don't work on your tendon and ligament strength in the first two phases, you could get some bad injuries. Also, if you don't work on your muscle recruitment in the first phase, you will not utilize all the muscles you should to give the optimal power output without over-fatiguing you muscles quickly.

Like I said earlier, running is a power exercise that is hard on the body. Power exercises are like running times three. These exercises are very hard on the body, and if done too often, may cause great physical and mental fatigue. These movements generally use all of your lower body muscles and all your core muscles. You should generally do power exercises one time a week; maximum, two times. Strength and stability training should take place the other one to two times you lift that week.

Although I do them these lifting workouts after races or hard track interval training, do them if you're too tired. This can put a fair amount of stress on your tendons and ligaments if your muscles are too fatigued. Go for a good cool down, get something with high sugar and easily absorbed protein, and then lift when you feel good and ready to do so.

You do not want to lift with the legs before workouts or on your easy days. If you do them before your workout, you can easily over-fatigue and ruin your running workout. And like I said earlier, running is the most important thing you can do to get better at running. You do not want to lift with your legs on an easy day before a workout or the day after a workout because your body won't have ample time to recover from the extreme stresses of the running workout. "Take your easy days easy, and your hard days hard," is a saying I agree with. Lifting with your upper body is fine on your easy days. I like to go for a base run or tempo run after my Navy Seal workout.

Power drills should be lessened when you're taking a down week in the middle of a season. Strength and stability work can be done on down weeks, but to maximize recovery of your mind and body, I would not do many power drills. Doing one long set of power drills is fine. The max I'll do is three sets of two different exercises, but I generally won't do any other power drills after that set.

Otherwise, I generally pick seven to ten running specific power drills to perform once each. I generally do them across the entire infield of an outdoor track. They are extreme impact drills so you generally want a very soft surface so you don't tear up your feet. My favorite is doing them barefoot on the fake grass football fields. You know, the ones with ground tires for the dirt, Astroturf, if you will. You can't beat that surface for power drills.

Exercises

Squat

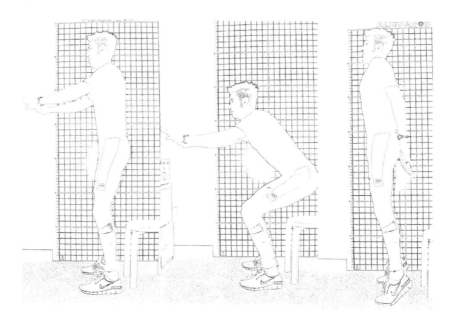

This is one of the most important exercises for a runner. It directly works out your prime mover and core muscles, and teaches your muscles to fire correctly and work together. It also strengthens you bones, ligaments, and tendons that take a harsh beating on the roads and track. Any muscle developed from this exercise (gluteus maximus, quadriceps and hamstrings), will not hurt the runners running performance at all. And if done in high sets and reps like I recommend, they should only tone and strengthen. Plus running 50 plus miles a week ought to keep mid to long distance runners leg from bulking up and looking like a sprinter's. I do tons of squats, lunges, etc and I can wrap my hands around my quads... kind of sad.

Focal Points:

1. KEEP KNEE OVER HEEL!!!!! Be a stickler, a Type-A personality, the no-exceptions kind of person on this one; it's very important for

knee health. If your knee comes in front of your toe or behind your heel on a squat or lunge you are putting most of the weight on your knee joint. This is bad. You want all the weight on your muscles and you want to indirectly strengthen your joints. All the weight goes straight down from where ever you have your knee at when pushing yourself back up. If nothing is there, all the weight is on your joint, if you have your heel under it, there is no bad joint pressure. If you let your knee buckle in or bow out you will have the same effect. And eventually, you will die. Okay, you won't, but your knees will hate you.

Football players blow out their knees by letting their knees come too far forward on this exercise. And while you may not be doing as much weight, you can wear down your knees, and generally when you hear somebody say, "I don't squat or lunge because it hurts my knees." It's because they are doing it wrong. I had a 75-year-old man with a torn MCL do a lunge and squat with no pain when he did it correctly. Pain was there when his knee came forward. But if he could do it without knee pain, you can too. So watch yourself in a mirror, or have somebody watch you on this one to make sure your knee does not come forward. Even if it doesn't hurt now if you're doing it wrong, add time and weight and you will eventually have some knee problems. Remember: KNEE OVER HEEL!!!

2. Rotate your hips back and tuck in your lower back. Basically stick yo butt out! Like a peacock showing off his tail feathers, or like you're taking a crap in the woods. This helps you utilize more glutes in the movement, which is where your stride should originate from, and stabilizes you knee better. It also aligns your spine so you don't get lower back pain if you have weight on your shoulders. This is also correct running form, so the more you practice it in the weight room, the more naturally you'll be able do it on the track. I'll go over running form in a bit too… don't worry.

3. Head up, chest out. You should be able to see the ceiling the entire time through the movement.

4. Counter balance yourself, push through your heel, not your toes at the deepest part of your squat. You want to reach your arms

forward and put your chest on you quad while sticking your butt up and keeping your head up. This allows you to push through your heels when you are down low.

5. Go down to a little above a 90-degree angle in your legs. Some trainers want a 'full Range of Motion' for squats and want you to go deeper than a 90, but what normal everyday activity does anybody do where they load their legs dipping below a 90 degree? I think this is bad for your knees as well, (lot of torque) so make sure not to go any lower than a 90 degree in your legs; I never get that close to a 90 because I have VERY bad knees ever since I was a young lad. But they're fine now!

6. When you are near the top it's okay to push with your forefoot onto the ball of your foot; I recommend it. This allows you to strengthen the muscles in the correct sequence that your muscles should work while running. This will help if you have an "under active" muscle, which is basically when your muscle doesn't fire in the right order and you get injured because of it. I find runners generally have under active glutes more so than anything else, and I know this exercise helps that problem.

A chair could help form at the start since this is how most people sit down and get up in a chair. You don't have to use the chair after you have the form down, but at the start it's nice to have there to feel correct form. You might feel off balance at first or like you're going to fall backwards and may even think you look like a new-born giraffe on ice. That's all right, perfection does not come instantly, but only through passion and desire mixed with knowledge.

Different Stances
There are three different stances that you can use while performing a squat and each stance will work different muscles.

1. *Feet together facing forward.* Same focal points on all the stances. This will work on the outside quad/Iliotibial Band a little more.

2. *Feet shoulder width apart facing forward.* This will work on your mid-quad/gluteus maximus more.

3. *Feet wider than shoulder length, facing 45-degree angle away from your body.* This will work on your inner quad/groin more.

Periodizations

1. *Stability:* do all the stances on a Dyna disc, airex pad, half of a foam roller, wobble board, or anything else that will make you focus and strive to hold a perfect center of gravity going through the movement. You can be creative, but please don't do something stupid and blame me. But if you do, send me the story, I love funny stories. Do 2 sets of 15 to 20 reps, but make sure you're concentrating and using all the little muscles in your legs to keep yourself balanced. Speed and weight is not important in this phase.

2. *Muscle Endurance:* Add dumbbells in your hands or weight on your back/shoulders. Do at least 20 reps for 3-6 sets. You should be a little more stable by this point, but still focus on form. It is always important, especially with weight. Go pretty quick through this, as fast as you can with good form.

3. *Power:* Same focal points, but initially push through the heel, then through the toes as you leap off of the ground. Land soft on your toes then to heels going all the way back down. You should not make much noise on this movement. Go as quick as possible and get as high as possible. You can have weight in your hands or on shoulders for this one, but you don't necessarily need it. Do anywhere from 20 - 30 reps for 2 - 3 sets.

Leg Press

The leg press is very similar to the squat, just less stability muscles are needed in it. Follow the same focal points as the squat, keeping knees over heels and not letting them bow in or out are the main ones to remember. For this one you can push with your midfoot a little more than the squat, but still focus on pushing mainly through your heels, especially when your knees are bent the most. This one is nice if you don't want to think too much through the workout. Breathe out when you are exerting force, and in when you are exerting less force to go back to the start position. Remember to breathe for every exercise.

Periodization
1. *Stability:* This really isn't a stability exercise.
2. *Muscle Endurance:* This is the king of muscle endurance exercises in my book. You can focus a little less on form and a little more on sets, reps speed and weight. I like to do around 300 – 400lbs 20 times with 3 - 6 sets. Do not start out that high!! Work your way into it, again, keep the sets and reps high all the time, and gradually move up in weight. You'll be very sore after your first time regardless of the weight, may as well not obliterate yourself first time out. There will be other times to do that.
3. *Power:* This really isn't a power exercise either... you could turn it into one if you want by lowering the weight significantly and pressing the weight up as fast as possible. But the key for power movements is teaching all your muscles to recruit together to optimize your power per stride and equal your disbursement of energy usage in your leg muscles. This will not do that for you because you're in a machine. So like corduroy and bell-bottoms, I highly recommend not doing it. Squat jumps are better.

Lunge

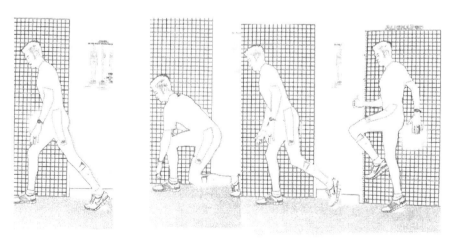

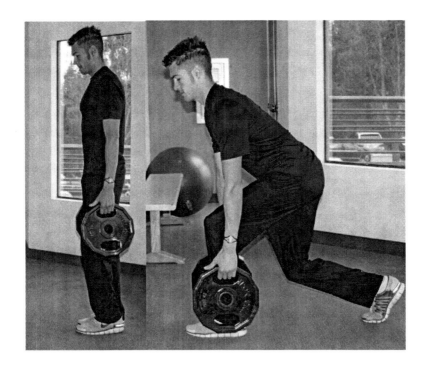

This is another great prime mover exercise for your legs. And one that is often done incorrectly and consequently, people generally have knee problems from doing this one wrong as well. But nonetheless, El Guerujji's main muscle endurance workout consisted of lunges and squats. So I feel they are very important as well.

Focal Points
1. KNEE OVER HEEL!! This one is probably worse than the squat for people frequently letting their knee move too far forward on a lunge. Keep it directly over your heel, for the same reason I stated earlier.
2. Hips rolled back, butt out, and lower back tucked in. If they feel it in their quads they might not be doing this part correctly. Or they might be pushing through their toes in the lowered position and are

not pushing through their heel. Push through the heel while you're low and toes while you're high in the position.

3. Put your chest on your thigh to put all the weight on your front foot. You should again counter balance yourself so you can push through your front heel, and not with your back toe. If you push yourself forward with your back toe while doing a lunge it will cause knee and quad pain in your trail leg. For that reason, you have to lean forward enough to put all the pressure through your front heel so you won't use your back leg at all during the lunge. I like to pick up my back leg as I start to come up from a lunge. It helps your balance at the same time and insures you don't push off of your back toe.

4. And for the same reasons I stated in the squat, I sometimes put my knee in the air and do a single leg calf-raise to finish the lunge; it's great for working your stability muscles.

Stances

You can step forward and walk, reach one leg back and bring it up again, step 45 degrees to the side with each leg, or even sideways. Being a single leg movement you are going to incorporate more muscles in the movement than a double leg movement (squat or leg press), so it's not a necessity at all. I don't really see much benefit to doing it all different ways, but there might be people out there who would tell me I'm wrong.

Periodization

1. *Stability:* You really don't need to do anything special for this phase. Just don't add any weight and do them right. It will be awkward enough if you've never done them before or done them correctly. But it will come around with practice. And you'll know when you can move to the next phase, when it ain't no thang to keep your balance.

2. *Muscle Endurance:* I like to hold onto dumbbells during this phase, or plates with handles. I currently hold a 35lb plate in each hand and do 3 - 4 sets of 20 lunges each leg. But when you're just getting started, keep building up the weight and keep reps and sets

high. Keep good form but get through it quick or you'll be here all day on this one.

3. *Power:* I normally do jump lunges for this one with no weight. Start off in proper lunge position, push through the heel then toe as you're about to leap up, try not to use your back foot that much at all in this, but it might be inevitable. Get as high as you can and switch feet in the air landing on your opposite foot as soft as possible. Repeat as quickly as you can.

Step Up

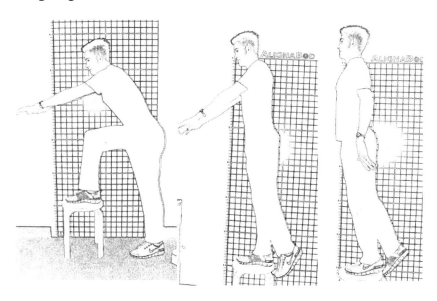

This is very similar to the lunge and works out the same muscles in a different way. It is a bit more difficult than a lunge but is a very good substitute. You can do this one on bleachers, or stairs if you have a large group of athletes and not enough step-up boxes.

Focal Points

*Focal points for a step up are very similar if not pretty much the same as a lunge.

1. Start off with your chest on your quad that's up on the box. This will put all your weight on your front leg and allow you to push through your heel and not your back leg. If you have to use your back foot, you're either not strong enough to do this yet or you're not leaning far enough forward at the start.

2. Keep back foot dorsi flexed (pull your toes off the ground). This will ensure that you do not use your back leg.

3. Stand all the way straight up before you go back down keeping your same leg up there. Don't let your other foot touch until it reaches the ground softly; do not let it fall fast and hard. And do not rock off the ground with your back foot.

4. Like the lunge and the squat, you can add a calf raise at the end to go through the chair if you would like. Again, this works your stability muscles.

Periodization

1. *Stability:* Just getting the form right without weight is plenty to keep your motor skills active and your brain neurons doubling. Once you are confident on the form you can add weight, but you will be sore from this one with no weight; it is very difficult.

2. *Muscle Endurance:* You really don't need weight for this one ever, but I have added upwards of 45 lbs stepping up onto a bench press bench. I normally do this 12 - 15 times each leg 1 - 2 sets.

3. *Power:* This is a great power exercise; a bench might be too high for most people to really develop their power on this exercise. I would recommend doing it on a lower platform for newbies. Explode off your front leg, get as high as possible with control, land soft, and use your back leg as little as possible. Repeat as quickly as you can. I like to do 1 - 2 sets of about 20 reps each leg on this one.

Single Leg Glut Bridge

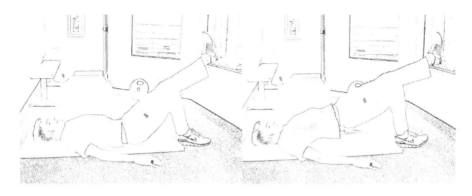

This is similar to the leg press in that it's not good for stability or power, but is a great muscle endurance exercise that you don't have to think as much about. This is a great exercise for an under active gluteus maximus. This is your athlete with hamstring issues. Get them on this one OFTEN. It will be a panacea for the bum hamstring masses.

This movement is performed on your back with one foot close to your gluts, right under your knee (not too far out and not to far in). While the other is held straight in the air, parallel to your other thigh with no movement. You push down through your heel of the foot on the ground and lift your pelvis off of the ground until your body's straight, then lower down and repeat. Remember, the leg you have up in the air should not move.

Focal Points
1. Keep hands at your sides and back flat on ground. Keep one foot flat, heel under knee. Keep the other leg straight out with thighs parallel and unmoving throughout the entire movement.
2. Push through heel, not toe.
3. Focus on Gluts while performing exercise to ensure that you are using them the most. Sounds stupid but it works!

Periodization

Like I said earlier, this is really only a muscle endurance exercise. I like to do 3 - 4 sets of 25. But sometimes I'll just do one set of 50. You can rocket through these too, but make sure you go all the way up and all the way down. This is a good substitute for lunges and step-ups if you're sick of them, but the other two are better to do more often.

Abductor and Adductor Planks with Dip

This is a great exercise for people with weak Iliotibial (IT) bands, bad knees, and runners with a large sway from side to side.

Abduction:

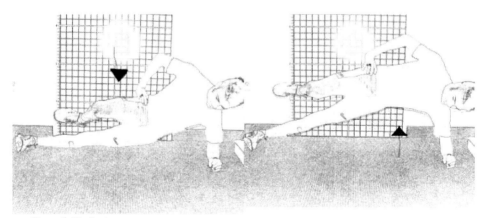

Focal Points
1. Lay on side, elbow on ground, and leg straight.
2. Lift your leg that's on top in air up so it does not touch your leg that's on the ground at all.
3. Push hips up in the air from the side of your foot. Keep your butt in line with shoulders and your foot on the ground with your elbow.
4. Do not let ankle buckle. This will work on your ankle stability as well.
5. Focus on your IT band as you bring your hips up and down.

Adduction

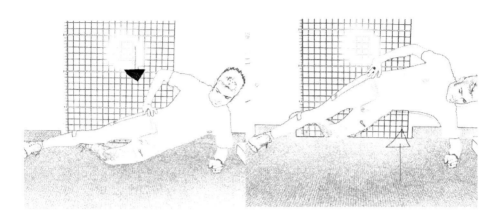

Focal Points

1. Same position but this time your leg that was in the air is the one with the side of your shoe cushion on the floor. And the leg that was on the floor is tuck in the air underneath the side of your body.
2. Move your hips up and down touching your hips and dangling leg on the floor. Focus on your groin muscle.

This could be a stability or muscle endurance exercise. I generally only do one set of 20 for these guys to add to my stability or muscle endurance routines. I prefer the machine you sit in and move your legs out and in, but since most people won't have that lying around, this is a great alternative that works more muscles than the machine.

Straight planks

Straight planks are a common and really good core workout. I learned recently a great way to strengthen core stability muscles for runners. Lifting up one elbow and putting it down then same with other arm, keep your hips motionless. It's very difficult at first. Spread your legs wider at the start, this makes it easier. As you get better you can put them closer together. You can also do this on your hands with straight arms. Focus every time to keep hips from moving.

Leg Swing

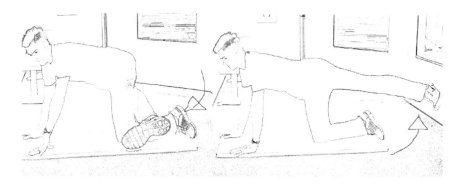

This is a great one to use for band IT bands and non-firing Glutes. You might make fun of people you see doing this exercise at the track, but it is one of the best you can do to keep you Lower Pelvic Hip Complex healthy and firing correctly.

Focal points

1. Start on the floor on all four. Keep your back flat. I want to be able to eat off of it, and Heaven help you if you spill my red wine!
2. Keep one knee on the ground and straighten out your other leg so it's parallel with the floor off the ground. Keep both hands on floor.
3. Keep foot turned sideways so your toes are pointing towards the horizon, and dorsi flex your toes the whole time.
4. Move your leg as far back as you can, keeping it sideways. Then kick it forward as close to your shoulder as possible keeping it sideways and straight the whole time.
5. Keep you core contracted the whole time; do not let your body sway with your foot.

Periodization

This is solely a muscle endurance exercise, but one of the best. I like to do 20 - 30 of these then do kick backs, which is very similar but you bend your knee and kick your foot back keeping it sideways. I kick back 20 - 30 times then do the other leg and call it a day. Sometimes I add 5lb weights to my legs with these, but it's all ready pretty hard, and most of the times I'd rather just add more reps.

Leg Lift

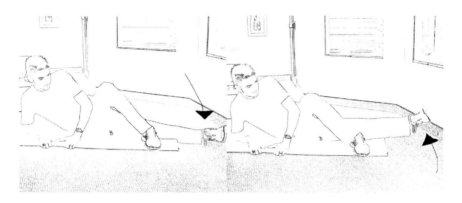

This one is good if you do not have a gym or do not want to do the planks. It's a good way to effectively strengthen your groin /abductor without too much effort, thinking, or equipment. Putting a 5lb weight on the end of your leg is a bit more effective if you have it though. Or maybe you could just wear a pair of boots instead.

Focal Points:
1. Lay on your side, elbow on ground, and bottom leg straight.
2. Put other leg over the leg on the ground so that your foot is in front of knee.
3. Lift the bottom leg as high as you can off of the ground and then lower.
4. Repeat 30 – 50 times both sides.

Three Way Calf Raise and Bent Knee Calf Raise.

These are CRUCIAL for a runner's health. Keeping your calf and Achilles tendon healthy can be an arduous task if you do you have a proper weight routine. I cannot tell you how many runners have been sidelined because of these two muscles.

Calf Raise

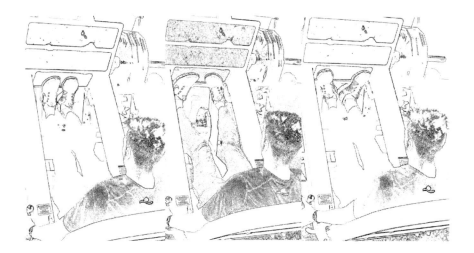

Focal Points
1. Keep legs and body straight the entire time with only your foot joint changing angles.
2. Make sure your toes are the only things touching the platform, and that your heels have enough room to lower down as far as your calves will stretch comfortably.
3. Go quick but try not to bob the weight. A slight pause each direction change will take care of this.

Periodization
1. *Stability:* Do single leg calf raises without touching anything. If that's too easy, close your eyes and try it. Do only 1 or 2 sets of 25 to 30 reps.

2. *Muscle Endurance:* I like to rack up the weight on the leg press for this one and crank 'em out doing all directions 20 times each way in 2 sets. I start and finish with straight feet so it's a totally of 80 calf raises with a fair amount of weight. But you can do them with dumbbells, or on a squat machine with weight is also very good.

3. *Power:* Don't go all directions for this one; just do straight legged hops or jump rope with straight legs the entire time for good calf power. I don't really think it'd be a good idea to try a power drill for your Achilles. It takes too much of a beating just running. Hills are a good Achilles power workout, too much and you'll get tendonitis though.

Bent Knee Calf Raise (Achilles)

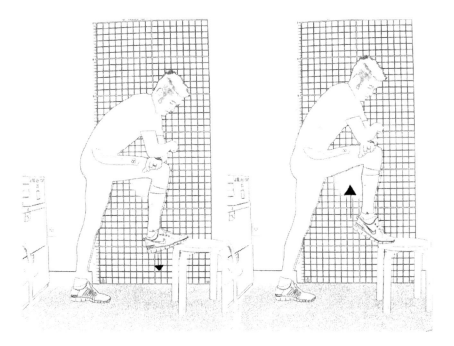

Focal Points

1. Put one leg up on a box or two stairs up with only your toes and the ball of your foot on the platform.

2. Keep your knee bent at about a 90 degree angle and lock it in that position for all of the movement.

3. Keep your knee over your heel.

4. Lean on your leg on the platform and put as much body weight as possible on the leg doing the calf raise. You can also put a weight on your knee instead.

5. Move your heel up and down focusing on your Achilles.

Stances

1. Point toes in and heels out with the movement to focus on the outside of your calf or Achilles.

2. Point toes straight forward to work on the bed of the Gastrocnemius or Achilles

3. Point toes out and heels in to work on the inside calf or Achilles.

*Note: This only works for the Achilles if you have a bent knee calve raise machine. If you can only do one foot at a time, you will have to move your foot in a rainbow type arch to hit all your sides if you can't do both feet at once. Move your heel as far as you can to the left, and then go as high as you can, moving it to the right as you go. Keep your knee still.

Single Leg Stabilization (Dyna disc)

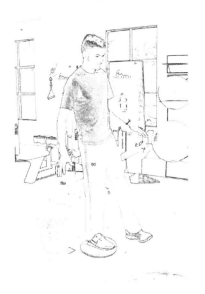

   This exercise is for the weak of ankle. If you have ever sprained your ankle or are afraid you're going to, this is the exercise for you. When you sprain you ankle you pull all the ligaments and tendons and they become stretched out and weak. This makes you very susceptible for another sprain or worse injuries for a very long time after the incident. The absolute best way to recover fast and strengthen all your tendons and ligaments after a sprain is to hop on a Dyna disc. This is that little squishy rubber pad that you always wondered what in the world it was for in the weight room. There are also wobble boards, half foam rollers, airex pads, and bosu balls (single leg upside down bosu ball is one of my favorite ankle strengthening exercises). If you can't find any of these, try just standing on one foot, closing your eyes, and moving in different ways trying to lose your balance while at the same time trying stabilizing yourself with your ankle. This is also good for Achilles tendinitis, but not as good as the bent knee calf raise.

Focal Points
1. Stand on one leg, straight, with no bend in the knee on a Dyna disc.
2. Stay on it for one or two minutes each leg.
3. If you don't feel it in your ankle, your knees might be bent or you should try making it more difficult by trying to lose your balance a little more.

This is mainly a stabilizing exercise but can be added to any workout, especially if you have bad balance.

Toe Raise

This is a must for the shin-splinted runner. You have micro tears in your muscles that are not healing very fast and running does not help the situation. As a runner you can either take a lengthy time off and hope it doesn't happen again or you can strength train your shin; recovering it much faster, and dramatically reducing the risk of it happening again. This will make it hurt worse initially, like I talked about earlier, you have to break it down to build it up, and so that's a good thing. Keep going! For this exercise you sit down on stair and let your toes hang off the edge of the stair beneath you. Put some weight on you shoes evenly dispersed and lower your toes and then lift them as high as possible afterwards. Wash, rinse and repeat.

Focal Points
1. Make sure the weight doesn't hurt your foot
2. Focus on your shin while pulling it up. If you don't feel it working that's probably part of the problem, your brain isn't firing it correctly. Give it time; your brain will come around.
3. Knees over heels.

I normally put a 45 lb plate on my toes and lift it up and down until my shins are completely fatigued. I only do one set of these though. You don't need to do as much with the smaller muscles, but you do need to do something. In all honesty, you do not need weight on your toes to fatigue your shins. Just lift you toes as high as they will go and keep going until your shines are fatigued. It shouldn't take long. You can do it while listening in class, watching a movie, or even when getting a lecture from the parents! It's a beautiful thing.

Shin splints probably have something to do with your running form as well. A lot of runners tend to pull their toe up while their foot is in the air because of excess heel padding; this can easily over fatigue the shine muscle. Keep your foot relaxed and hanging down close to the ground while bringing it forward, I'll go over this more later.

Bound

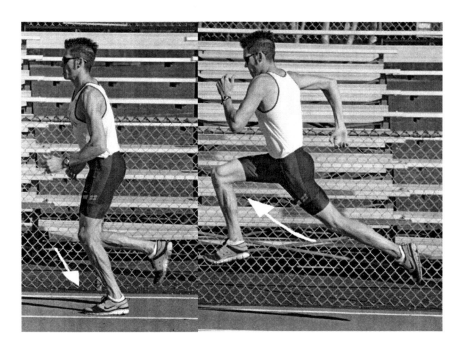

This is probably the most sports specific power movement you will find. It mimics your running stride the most and if done correctly can increase your power per stride the most. This is the one sole power exercise I will go over because it's the most important.

Others that I like are include High Knee Skips, Box Jumps, Straight Leg Bounds, Straight Leg Shuffle, Single Leg Hop, Side Shuffle Bound, Hurdle Jumps, and Frog Leaps are all ones I dabble in now and then on a power routine day. But the Bound is always first and considered my most important. You should look goofy during this one, so be prepared. But you just make gawkers look goofy be kicking their butt around the track.

Focal Points
1. Get a running start for momentum.
2. Land on the ball of your foot slightly behind your body driving it down hard and fast leaping as far as possible from that one bound.
3. Drive the other leg up in the air hard with your opposite hand and hold your knee there as long as you can in a 90 degree angle before driving it down to start your next bound. The goal is to keep that leg up in the air longer and longer. This means you're going further and developing more power per stride.

I generally go the whole length of a football field; I can cover the field in about 12 bounds (24 steps or so), so I generally go back for another length. The goal is to try to keep shortening your number of strides per football field as you progress. But remember, power is strength times speed, so without doing your strength work you will not get that much power. Also, you don't want to start out doing an exercise like this without prepping your ligaments, tendons, and muscles first. That's a good way to end up in the training room. This exercise is far harder on your legs than running is, so I would be careful with how often you do it. Respect the drill, it can make you faster but it can also contribute to injuries. Using it properly is a wonderful addition to any running program.

High Knee Skips

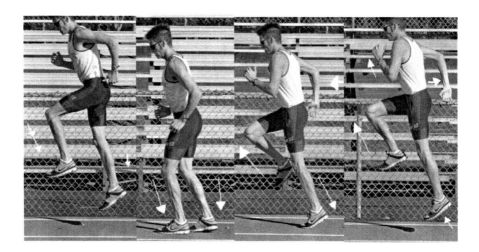

This is similar to the bound but it is more vertically based. For this one you go up more than out. This is another good power drill for runners. Along with the bound it teaches symmetry with your body and works all the same running muscles with more force/impact/power.

Focal Points
1. Bring one knee up and opposite arm as hard as you can controlled and jump up like you're skipping.
2. Hold that position while in the air.
3. As you come down, drive the foot higher in the air down fast so it strikes at the same time as the other leg.
4. As you bound back up with that harder striking foot, lift up the other leg high and hard and repeat the process.
5. Get as high as you can each time.

This is a good one to do after the bound. Do the bound first since it's the most taxing. This is good to do around 20 times each leg. Again, a soft surface is good for all these drills.

Lower Back

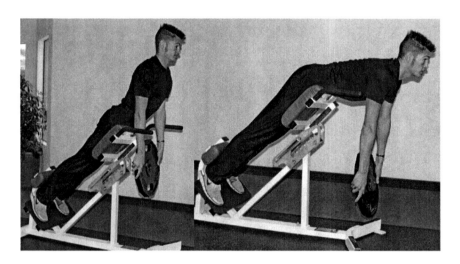

This can be a problem for most runners if not strengthened. If you cannot hold your spine in correct form for the duration of your race, then you will have lower back pain from you bones taking all the impact and not dispersing it properly. Some runners develop stress fractures in their lower back due largely impart to the muscles are too weak around that area. My favorite way to strengthen my lower back is on the back extension machine, holding a 45lb plate, dipping down 40 times in 3 sets. Keep your head up or you will get a head rush from all the blood going to your head. If you do not have a back extension machine you can do sky divers.

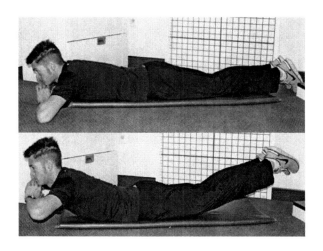

Focal Points
1. Lay on stomach comfortably.
2. Place hands under chin to support neck during exercise.
3. Arch your shoulders and your feet as high as possible balancing on your abs so you look like the latter U.
4. Focus on your lower back throughout the movement.

This one is good because you can do it anywhere. I like to do these at varied paces and some times I hold for around five seconds arched as high as I can. But I'll generally get in at least 50 reps in 2 to 6 sets.

Routines

Now that you know how to perform all the basic movements you need to help out your running routine, I'm going give you tips and even some routines that have been effective for me and have had a great deal of thought put into them. I am a gym rat, so I do put a lot of thought into this stuff, I promise.

The first thing you need to know is order. It's best to workout your larger muscle groups first and the most; then the smaller muscle groups after but not as much. This way, your smaller muscle groups can help you with form better throughout your workout, and you can workout your larger muscle groups more effectively. Also, as you get tired, it's easier to work on smaller muscles at the end of workouts. Basically the closer to the belly button the muscle, the larger it's going to be and the more important it is to work them out first. Abs, lower back, and obliques can be worked out at any time, or throughout the entire workout. Some routines that I set up have some things in them that I did not cover, but they are very easy to learn and there's little risk of injury. Just don't ever start off with tons of weight on anything at the start. Common sense is the moral of the story.

Stability Routine

- 3 Way Squats on Dyna discs. (Feet together, shoulder width apart, and further out point 45 degrees out) 20 each way X 1 or 2 sets.
- 3 x 12 step up
- 3 x 30 skydivers
(I'll do these three exercises in a row times three as fast as possible before moving on to the next)
- Cable leg abduction and adduction, all 4 ways, 20 times each, normally only 1 - 2 sets
(the bobbing side planks would work here too; I talked about earlier)

- single leg calf raise without holding on to anything else, 25 - 50 each leg, only 1 set
- bent knee calf raise, 25 - 50 each leg, only 1 set.
- single leg Dyna disc balance, one minute on each leg, no touching.
- finish with abs, back and oblique exercises, call it a day.

Muscle Endurance Routine

- Squats with weight or leg press, 3 - 6 sets of 20 reps. I like to do around 300lbs and move up to 410lbs in the machines.
- Lunges with weight, 3 - 6 sets of 20 reps each leg. I like to do around 60 - 80 lbs
- Back extension, 3 - 5 sets of 30 to 50 reps. I'll do around 45 - 55 lbs
(I do these three together as fast as possible before moving on)
- Leg swings, 2 sets of 20
- Groin and IT band up and down bridge, 2 set of 20
(I normally do adductor/abductor machine for this one back to back)
- Calf raises, 3 way plus 1 more straight forward, 20 each (80 total), 1 or 2 sets. I do around 250 - 300 lb for this one on leg press of squat machines.
- Bent knee calf raise. 3 plus 1 way times 15 (60 total), 70 to 90 lbs. 1
- 2 sets (If no machine I use a 50 - 60lb dumbbell one leg at a time. Or just put as much of my weight as possible on my knee doing the movement)
- Ab and oblique exercises to follow. I know you know tons of ab workouts. Mix it up, make them burn.

Muscle Endurance Routine #2

- Leg Press, 2 x 30. I do around 250 lbs
- Step Ups, about 15 each leg with 50 - 60 lbs, 1 set (do in-between leg press sets)
- Back Extension, 100 reps no weight times 2 (put the 2nd set somewhere else in the workout)

- Leg Extension machine, 4 sets of 15 - 20 reps. I do around 155 - 175 lbs
- Leg Curl machine, 4 sets of 15 - 20 reps. I do around 110 - 130 lbs (Super set these two exercises, back to back times four)
- Single Leg Glute Bridge, 3 x 25 each leg
- Adductor/Abductor machine 2 x 30 each way.
- Calf Raises and Bent Knee Calf Raises same as previous set
- Balance on dyna disc or airex pad
- Five or six minutes of non-stop abdominal exercises. Keep switching it up when too tired; try to get close to 300 reps.

Power Routine

- Bound, 25 times each leg
- Hurdle jumps (or rocket jumps, box jumps or frog hops) 30 times in a row
- High knee skips, 25 times each leg
- Straight legged bound, 25 times each leg
- Straight legged shuffle, 60 times each leg as fast as possible.
- Side bound, 20 each way
- Single leg hop. 15 each leg

Mix Power and Muscle Endurance routine

- 24 deep lunges
- 12 deep jump lunges
- 24 step back lunges (or normal if you prefer)
- 12 jump lunges

Go through this as fast as you can, take a 30 second break and do it 2 - 4 more times. No weight needed.... trust me.

These are about the only routines I generally use. I switch them up a little all the time, but that's the basics of them and they have worked wonders for my running and injury prevention. Once you know the basics, you can develop your own personal workout routine that you like. Just remember the basics and you'll be all right. Olympic lifts are arguably one of the best power movement exercises you can do (Snatch, Clean and variations), but they are too complex to give a great explanation of them. Plus there's a good possibility for injury if you do it wrong. My advice would be to go to a gym rat or guru and ask him to teach you and watch your form for you, or hire a good trainer like me. But this full body power movement is said to release the most HGH and Testosterone afterwards.

(All photos in this Lane were taken by Jerry Banks)

Lane 5

Form:
Strength wins High School; Efficiency wins Olympics

This section could have potentially been at the start of the science section. Form is a topic that is seldom discussed in running circles, but should be perfected by all coaches and runners. Some elite runners have awful form and they run phenomenally! And some of those runners that tried to change their form later ran worse with correct form so they never changed it. But OF COURSE you're going to run a little worse initially because you're not used to using those muscles in that way yet. Some times you have to take a step backward to move two steps forward though. The good news is that you can change it for the better; the bad news is that you will feel like a newborn giraffe on ice. Fight through it and keep getting better. Changing running mechanics to be more efficient will be better for a runner in the long run, no pun intended. But I do know that the most efficient runners have a higher performance ceiling than the in-efficient runner. This is probably why all the efficient runners have all the world records. Michael Johnson, Noah Ngeny, Hicham El Guerrouj, Daniel Komen, Kenenisa Bekele and one of my all-time favorites Sebastian Coe who broke numerous world record times in his carrier. And for you road warriors that don't think form matters off the track, watch Haile Gebrselassie's form while running a marathon. In this chapter I will try to put into words all of the little details that go into being an efficient and graceful runner. But the best way for you to learn is to watch some of the most efficient runners run and try to mimic them. Efficient runners are easy to pick out. They look like they're jogging when they're runner sub 60-second quarter pace. The best form I've ever seen was El Guerrouj, some people say different stuff about him but one thing you cannot deny is that he had amazing form and made 55 second pace look like a casual jog in the park. So if you really want to see great form, watch him. But here are a few things to get you started.

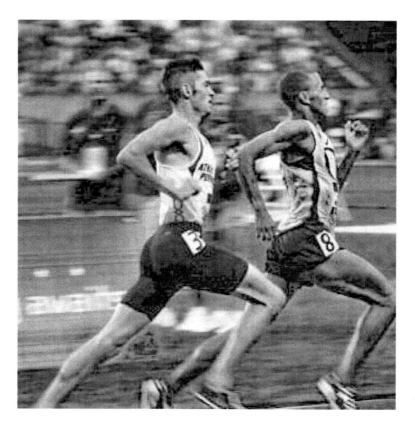

We'll start with the most important part, your foot strike. You should be landing on the ball of your foot, not on your heel or on your toe. You should be landing right underneath your hips at your center of gravity pulling your foot back. When you land on your heel you are working against yourself by stopping forward momentum landing in front of your center of gravity. If you lean slightly forward and land on the ball of your foot you will constantly be pushing backward working with your momentum. The only time I ever land on my heel is when I'm trying to stop myself going downhill, which I think is a great self-experiment to feel the efficiency different from forefoot running to heel running. Run down a slight downhill on your heels standing straight up and then go down the same hill running on your forefoot leaning slightly forward, landing right below your body or behind it. It will be like watching a basketball versus a football in a downhill race. Then you can have the final decision for yourself to see what the most efficient style is.

You're drive foot should be doing all the work while you're other foot being brought up should be relaxed. So relaxed that your toe hangs down when you're driving your knee forward **reflexively**. (Your other leg comes forward from basic reflexes, so working to bring it forward only uses more energy. I call this 'running in mud' because you're never relaxed.) This should make your toe point straight out when your leg is fully extended forward. Your toe should remain close to the ground through all of this phase. I call it the glide. This is like when swimmers practice keeping their hand close to the water. Your toe should be close to the ground. (Common mistake: runners tend to pull their toe up through the entire part of the running movement.) Watch for rocks and roots while off-roading. If you have very bad proprioception then maybe this is a bad practice for you. Or better yet, just learn to be aware of your surroundings. I can always tell the runners that don't have good proprioception. They bump around in the pack like a roller derby player... very annoying. Back to running form; a good practice to keep your toe low is to do the grass foot drag. Run through the grass and try to have your toe touch the grass the whole time while still landing on your toe. This at least lets you become more aware of where your toe is. If you cannot relax your foot through this movement then you will use a great deal more energy than you should be using. The runner will generally look like they're running through water or something like that when they use too much energy to get their foot forward. Also, they will typically bring their knee up and not forward if they strain to bring their foot forward. This will cause the use of a lot more energy and make you move more up and down instead of gliding across the track. It's your body's automatic response, so try not to do it.

After your toe has relaxed through the movement and is pointing straight ahead, it's time for that leg to do some work. Leading with your hip and butt, drive the knee back snapping your toe back quickly. This will snap your toe back quickly and should dorsiflex your toe so you land on your forefoot with your toe pulled up. This should make very little noise if done correctly. Since your toe was being pulled up as you were landing it should be a very soft landing and leave you landing slightly behind your center of gravity with a leg full of elastic potential ready to explode off of the ground. If you make a loud sound every step you take while running, you can bet your bottom dollar something is wrong with your form. Unless you're wearing clogs.

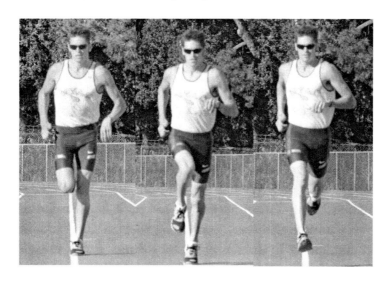

Along with landing on your forefoot, you should be landing in a straight line. I have my high schoolers practice running on the white lines of a track. If your feet land anywhere from symmetrically pointing straight forward to slightly in, that means you're symmetrical. This is also the most efficient way to run. I see many a duck foot running going on out there, and it needs to stop. Try watching a runway model walk down the line. Her hips might be flying on purpose, but she is landing in a straight line, and symmetry is beauty. (Although some of them step over the symmetrical line now-a-days, do not do this either... I only know this because my wife watches Project Runway!) Be symmetrical! I also have my high schoolers practice walking like a run way model so that running in a straight line seems more natural. This is something that you have to work on, because after the burden of life weighs on you, you get all out of whack. Fight it!

Roll your hips forward sticking your butt slightly out while running too. This aligns your lower back to give you a better push off and decrease lower back pain. Stand tall with your chest out but relaxed as well, basically, have good posture. Play with your hips rolling forward and back while you're just standing there to get a feel for good posture. If this is hard to do, work with weights on your lower back more; single leg glute bridges are essential. You should be able to maintain this posture throughout the entire day and while you're running. If you cannot, then it is a muscular problem that needs to be fixed in the weight room.

Your hands should be relaxed and staying symmetrical. I don't think it's a huge deal if they are high up on the chest or low, as long as you can keep them relaxed and fluid. You should always keep your hands as close to the body as possible. The further your hands are from your body the more energy is wasted, keep your hands close and relaxed. Wind milling is not acceptable. Keep your neck, shoulders and face relaxed. Your shoulders should not be rolled too far forward or it will be hard to stay symmetrical. They shouldn't be too far back either; keep them relaxed perfectly in the middle. Upper bodywork should help you keep form in this area. Keep a slight forward lean to make sure you land correctly. This will keep your body relaxed. Once you tense up, your brain will freak out and shut down your lungs and heart rate, the longer you can hold this off the faster you will run. You should slowly fall over with the forward lean if you were standing still. I have my kiddies start their strides sometimes by falling over forward to work on a slight forward lean. Occasionally you'll have one or two people bend over forward thinking they're leaning forward; not good. This will eventually cause lower back pain. You want their whole body in alignment when their foot is pushing off behind them. They will kick back after this point to slightly over extend they're leg. But this will enable them to effortlessly bring their foot back forward to strike back for the next stride. This means all the focus should be on the strike, and the leg will come back to start position without any energy or mental focus used to get it there. When people start rigging they tend to try and make their leg go through the entire movement, this only makes them go slower and use more energy. If they would jut focus on their push back they would go faster.

Some people say that you have to be going fast to have this perfect form, which means only strides and short races can have good form. This is a load of malarkey. I've done 11.5 second 100's with this form, I've done six-minute mile pace with this form, and I've done ten-minute mile recovery runs with this form. And all the people I talk to that have good form in all their races say the same thing, and have the same form in all their workouts and easy runs. This is generally an excuse used by people that don't want to try and work on their form so they say this so in their mind they justify their sloppy form. But it will show in a race.

A great way breathe and prevent asthma is by taking long deep breaths. The most common form of breathing for tired runners is mouth open, shallow, hyperventilating breathing like a panting dog. This is very bad for many reasons, namely: it will dry out your lungs faster causing asthma attacks, your blood will not oxygenate as much with shallow breathing, and the lack of pressure in your lungs will give the runner less blood pressure which means less power in your muscles. This is all very bad. The correct way to breathe while exerting maximal effort is taking a deep breath in and then blow through a slightly closed mouth keeping it in there a little longer. This is very important for people like me with sports induced asthma. Deep long breathing keeps the lungs moist longer for people like me that don't sweat very much. It also creates more slightly more pressure in your chest, which creates more blood pressure in your body, which then creates a greater maximal workload. During the kick phase of a race it's good to breathe out harder causing more pressure in the lungs creating more power for the last bit. Weight lifters call a similar technique a Valsalva Maneuver when they push air against their closed mouth to create move Blood Pressure to help lift a heavy object. This can cause too much blood pressure with a closed mouth and may pop blood vessels in your eyes giving you blood red eyes for a month or longer. This might be cool at Halloween, but for the other 364 days of the year it isn't; so don't do it. And finally, deep long breathing supplies more oxygen to your blood than quick shallow breathing, so like Big Red, you last a little longer.

One thing I do to try and get my high schoolers running more efficiently is running barefoot on the track for cool downs after workouts. This also strengthens your foot muscles that may be weak from high stability shoes that are marketed to runners with bad form… which is pretty much everybody. These shoes have ruined many a good runner and will continue to do so. Get out of them!! The less there is to your shoe, the better it is for you in the long run. Pun not intended because I don't like long runs. But anyways, feeling the ground more while running will help your brain recognize how it's landing better and should help you adjust your form a lot better. I think pain is the best teacher sometimes, and if you imagine running barefoot on rocks, you will not land on your heel or land hard. You would land very softly on your forefoot. This is probably why young kids that run around barefoot have great form, and then 5 years later after shoes it's awful.

There are probably a million other little things to get your form better. These are the bigger things that I have noticed help my form quite a bit. But there is always room for improvement and ways to improvement. Even a soccer ball rolled hard enough can out roll a basketball, but eventually with less force, the basketball will win. I encourage you to get out there and be a knowledge seeker in this area. Keep hammering out your form relentlessly until you feel like you're floating. You can always get better, so take your destiny in your own hands and do it.

Lane 6

Injury Prevention:
Can't Win if You Don't Get to the Line

Relax! Go to Sleep

A common problem with OCD runners is the inability to relax. When a runner is not running or racing they're thinking about the race or hard run that is coming up. Sometimes they even feel guilty for not running or working out in some way in their down time. This leads to too much stress and can ruin your health. One of the main things that this will do is increase the production of Cortisol and keep it in your system longer. This will hurt you in all the ways I talked about earlier when Cortisol is lingering in your system. When you have down time, let it be your down time. Let yourself be in the moment, enjoy it and relax. When you're running or training, be all about that. Don't let your mind wander to what you're doing that night, a song you like or anything else other than accomplishing your goal for that workout. The healthiest stage of your life is the infancy stage. In this stage of your life your heart rate sky rockets to 220 BPM and then goes right down to 30 BPM very fast. One of the leading markers in old age, obesity, depression, sickness, heart disease, cancer and diabetes is a monotonic heart rate. This is basically where your heart rate does not change rapidly or at all with different activities. The more you can lower your heart rate at rest the easier it will be to elevate during intense workouts and consequently the healthier you'll be and the faster you'll develop. In the words of a 9th grade philosophizing colleague, "Take a chill pill yo." (Ok don't really take a pill) Or maybe, "Don't worry, be happy."

Another thing that prevents recovery and ruins many a good runner is a lack of sleep. So how much sleep is enough? Well on average people need about 7 – 10 hrs of uninterrupted sleep. An elite athlete might need more to recover, but at least 8.5 hrs I'd say. A good way to find this out is to go to sleep and see what time you get out of bed naturally. If you could do this three to five days in a row and take the average it will be more accurate. How do you know if you're not getting enough sleep? Well, I Wikipedia's sleep deprivation to give you all the physiological effects, which are: *Aching muscles, blurred vision, cardiovascular disease, clinical depression, colorblindness, daytime drowsiness, decreased mental activity and concentration, depersonalization, weakened immune system, dizziness, dark circles under eyes, fainting, general confusion, hallucinations, hand tremors, headache, hernia, hyperactivity, hypertension, impatience, irritability, lucid dreaming, memory lapses or loss, nausea, nystagmus (rapid involuntary rhythmic eye movement), psychosis, pallor, slowed reaction time, slurred and/or nonsensical speech, weight loss or gain, severe yawning, suppresses growth hormones, inability to heal wounds, cramping, muscle fascia tears, reduces body's ability to metabolize glucose and is similar to being drunk.* (Wikipedia) I don't know about you, but getting an appropriate amount of sleep had me at the thought of "dark circles under your eyes," … yikes. Don't even come hear me with those, I will throw a pillow at you! And there are plenty of other symptoms to ruin a good runner. Pretty much every negative thing in the world will happen to you if you don't get sleep is the moral of the story. One of the more important things for an athlete to know is that Growth Hormone production is at its maximum during stage 4 sleep, Slow Wave Sleep. You should view your bed as your Super-Recovery-Adaptation-Re-energizing Chamber of Life! (SRARCoL©) Put a sticky note with that name on it above your bed. It will help you turn down the volume of 'urgent' issues but not 'important' ones from taking away your SRARCoL© time. Getting one less hour of sleep per night for seven days is just like staying awake for twenty-four hours once a week and you cannot make it up in one night. But you can play catch up; do it by going to sleep earlier, not sleeping in longer. To maximize your body's physiological and mental functions you need sleep. You can have an amazing training system with a great diet, but if this area is not under control it will all be for not.

"There is no hope for a civilization, which starts each day to the sound of an alarm clock." ~Author Unknown

http://en.wikipedia.org/wiki/Sleep_deprivation

Hip Alignment

Thee single most common problem that I have seen across all runners I have ever met is Hip Alignment Issues. If a part on one leg hurts and not on the other, it's almost always hip alignment. I've seen this with single sided hip, knee, hamstring, Achilles, calf and sometimes shin pain. Mainly knee pain is the first sign. If you run too long on a misaligned hip, you will get injured, typically on the foot taking more impact from the shorter leg. Do not let a doctor put a leg lengthening plastic insole on your shorter leg, this will only accentuate the problem. The best thing you can do is simply align your hips every time they go out. And it will happen often with track intervals, uneven roads, hills, and everyday use. It will go out less and less the more you align it. It's very easy to align your hips, you just have to do it. Here are the steps:
1. Lie on your back on a flat even surface.
2. Put knees up with feet flat on the ground symmetrically together.
3. Bring hips high off of the ground and lay it back flat on the ground to align your back.
4. Put your fist in-between your knees and squeeze your fist with you knees as hard as you can. You might feel a pop in your hips. This is good.

5. Put both your fist in-between your legs, and squeeze hard again.
6. Put your whole forearm in-between your legs and squeeze hard.
7. If you did not feel a pop in your hips and you don't feel better afterwards, try it again.
8. Do it again when the aggravated area hurts again. Do not run through the pain.

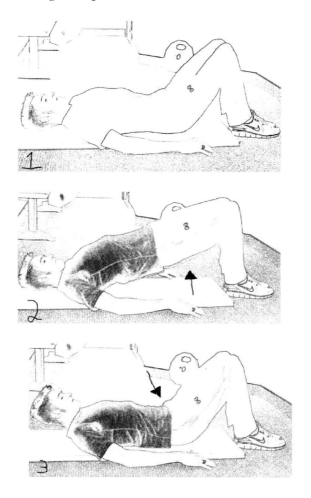

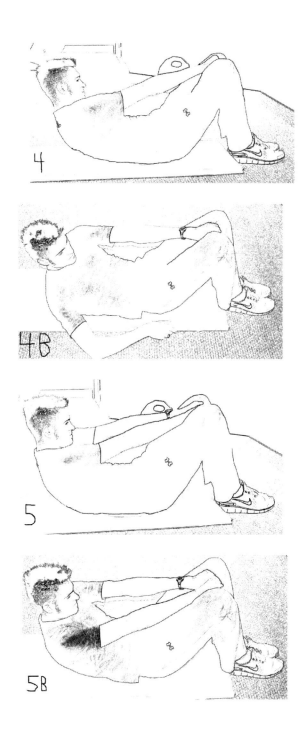

4

4B

5

5B

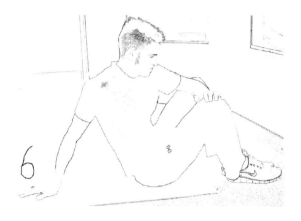

If your hips are rotated inwards, then you might want to try a very similar procedure to fix that. It's all the same as above except you push your knee up and the other knee down hard for a couple of seconds. Use your hands to keep them motionless but still try too move them as much as possible using your hips. If you have outside knee pain on one side, this can temporally relive it. But strengthening the hips and glutes will be the cure for this ailment.

This hip problem that can cause so many problems is normally cause by under active glute muscle, psoas, or other core muscle issues. To test out if you have this problem, sit down with your legs straight out in front of you. Rotate one leg as far as you can in and see if you can touch the floor. Then try the other leg and see which one cannot go as far as the other leg. The leg that cannot rotate as far in is the leg you have to work on to correct this problem. Do the same for rotating your leg outwards. Doing isometric leg holds should activate this muscle so it stops messing up your hips. Be careful, when I did this the first time because my hips were out, I was forced to use different muscles in the affected leg, which cause some muscle pulls. But after a while it went away and I didn't have to adjust my hips that much at all. And I utilized more muscles correctly in my stride... double bonus! So here's how you strengthen/activate that muscle group in your hip region:

1. Lay on your back with you legs straight out in front of you.
2. Rotate you toe that cannot twist inwards as much as the other leg as far as it's comfortable so it rests somewhere around the arch of the other foot.
3. Push the twisted foot into the other foot ever so slightly so you feel it in the outside of your glute muscle.
4. Hold the gentle push for six seconds, and repeat it six times. Do not push too hard or you will start to activate too many other muscles, namely your adductors, and not isolate the one you want to. You'll feel it.
5. Isometrically hold this 6 x 6 seconds pushing inwards, and then straight down the next set of 6 x 6 seconds.
6. Go the opposite direction for the other foot and do the same thing. You can work both sides with both legs, but focus on the one that's the weakest.

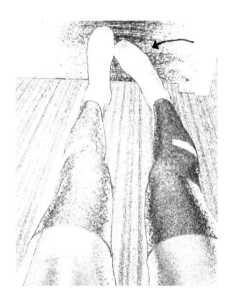

Normally if one foot cannot internally rotate better than the other foot, it can't rotate outwards as well. For this one it's best to do the same type of procedures as noted above except with your foot externally rotated. Push against the wall instead of your other foot though.

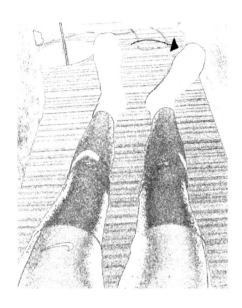

Another one you can use to activate an under active muscle in your knee is a bent knee toe push. This one is pretty similar to the one above except your knee is bent. I think when I tweaked my knee in the months prior to the Olympic Trials this exercise might have saved my butt. My last knee injury that was similar to this one took me out for over two months in high school. I have historically bad knees, even before running, so I think this exercise could help people like me. The bad knee was helped most by rotating the foot outwards. This seems to help the area where the IT band connects to the knee. Do the same sets as the one above, and don't push too hard. You can do both directions on this one too, but I don't find the one pushing in to help me personally that much.

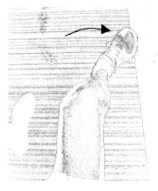

If these don't work for you, call the glue factory. Just kidding, but find a physical therapist that knows what he's doing enough to not prescribe drugs or ultrasound or anything other than strengthening you body to function correctly. They are out there, and that is how I learned. Find somebody that specializes in muscle energy. They will generally perform a few different tests to see if your strength in certain muscles is good. Frequently, the larger muscles will take over and then the smaller muscles will stop firing all together and cause numerous problems. The same person should be able to show you how to activate the muscles through simple touch or isometric exercises. If the therapist doesn't show you ways to activate the under active muscles, find another one.

Heat Treatment

I sort of laugh when I see all the runners freezing their butts off in a cold tub thinking it's going to make them recover faster. Maybe because this used to be me freezing my lower extremities off for 15 – 20 minutes. I'm not sure who started the rumor that cold is best for healing sports injuries, but man has it spread far and wide and people are religious about it. If I tell them cold might not be as effective for recovery as heat they almost take it personally, as if I had mocked their god. What this does is actually prevent healing and weaken your immune system. It prevents blood flow to the soar muscles, which prevents the healing process. Matthew Karl, MD, and Stanley Herring, MD, point out that the application of superficial heat to your body can improve the flexibility of your tendons and ligaments, reduce muscle spasms, alleviate pain, elevate blood flow, and boost metabolism. (1) The only time that it's recommended one should ice is when they just sprained their ankle or other joint and have localized swelling that could potentially further injure the joint. But I would argue that this could even be a mistake. What happens when you're running and you sprain your ankle? It swells up. But what happens if you sprain it, and keep on running? It doesn't swell up until you stop running. Why? This happens because the blood flow kept the swelling down. What happens when you ice? It does numb the pain, but it also constricts blood vessels making blood flow slow. It does reduce the swelling a little bit because of that, but since it's not good to ice too long it will swell up when you're done and keep it injured longer, even with habitual follow up icing. For a runner this is a negative thing. Your legs already have the worst circulation because they're furthest from your heart, making them the slowest healing area of your body. This is why your face heals from cuts in a few days, but your legs will take months to get rid of cut marks. But like external injuries, you want to increase your blood flow to the affected area, especially the areas further from the heart like you're feet. Have you ever noticed that when you get out of the Jacuzzi the blood vessels on your feet are swollen? This is the blood flowing action you want in your legs! This is also what makes a hot tub the best thing for tight, injured, soar and cracking joint feet. Heat also relaxes your body from the stresses of running, is better for the immune system, and just feels better in general. Heat rises moving the blood up more quickly from lower extremities. Cold goes down, making blood stay around longer in lower extremities. Cold is a vasoconstrictor, so it is good for stopping internal bleeding after an injury; I will give it that. Just about every other time, heat is better.

Another one I like to do is contrast. This is where you have your feet in cold water, then hot water for five minutes each. This rapid change in your legs environment can activate healing hormones to repair/rejuvenate your legs. I'm not sure if any research has been done on this, but it is just a theory of mine based on other things I know. Either way, the contrast therapy method is definitely one of the best and it's the only time I'll go in a cold pool. It also expands and contracts your blood vessels while keeping you blood flowing quickly. I do always end on the heat.

http://www.sportsinjurybulletin.com/archive/cold-therapy.html

NSAID's

These are Non-Steroidal Anti-Inflammatory Drugs. They suck. There is no need for these things, all they do is wreak havoc on your organs, prevent healing to injuries, reduce HGH and Testosterone/Estrogen in your body, which heals and recovers you, and most importantly, it masks the underlying issue causing the pain. Sometimes people take this for chronic muscle pain, but the pain is a message from your body that something is wrong and needs to be fixed. For these issues, the weight room is your best doctor. All most all runners will eventually have over active and under active muscles in their legs because of all the repetitions of strides a runner must take. Sometimes your muscles don't even fire in the right sequence causing added stress on certain muscles and giving you chronic pain in an area. It could even be a 'stress response' that is the precursor of a stress fracture. Both of which are saying, "Easy on the power stuff (running), we need some strengthening exercises (lifting)". Or it could be your hip is out of alignment, which I just talked about. But if it's any of these NSAID's will simply mask the underlying problem and make it harder to recover from. Even with a good weight room program NSAID's inhibit hormones that help you recover, reduce blood flow to prevent healing, and make it hard to know if you're making any progress. My advice, never take them. Especially the stronger ones... I have a personal Vendetta against those ones, but that's beside the point. Make your body stronger, don't just help it cope. It will be very hard to improve until you solve the underlying problem.

Stretching: Pro's, Cons, and Types

There are many things that one can say about stretching, so I will try to sum it up in one word: overrated. Stretching is not that beneficial for a runner. If you make yourself more flexible for a race by static stretching you will lose efficiency by making your tendons, ligaments and muscles more malleable. This will force you to use more muscle to go at the same pace, ultimately use more glycogen, and make you fatigue quicker. I do not do hard static stretching before a race or workout. I will do ballistic stretching. This gets your muscles used to movement while lengthening and contracting, which is much more sports specific. It allows your muscles to get used to the movement you're about to do so they do not get injured. Static stretching will not get you used to the movement you're about to do at all. Stretching really doesn't do much for the runner in general. If you stretch an injury you could pull the tendon/ligament worse than it already is, or tear the muscle more than it's already torn. It will also not increase blood flow or strengthen the affected area. Strengthening is what strength training will do for it without putting it past its Range of Motion (ROM) which would injure it further.

Physical therapists will tell you to "stretch more and ice", but if they tell you this, punch them in the face. Ok don't punch them in the face, but let them know in a cordial way that you need to be tight to perform at your best and you need blood flow. On average, people might think they need to be a little more flexible because if they slip or something it's a little easier to pull a muscle, tendon, or ligament. But in all honesty they're probably going to pull or tear it anyways if they fall badly enough. If people would workout their stability muscles a little more and quit buying bricks for shoes (heavy shoes for stability) to increase stability they might not get injured in this way as much. Or they think that the more Range of motion you have the longer your stride is. Don't listen to a therapist who got his knowledge in a classroom through a book written 20 years ago and makes money keeping you injured; use common sense, and instead listen to a guy who works on these injuries for a living and depends on his personal success in sport for his knowledge. Me. Ph D in life. I'll try to make that the last time I ever talk about myself in the third person... no promises. Exercise physiologists Mick Wilkinson and Alun Williams reach the same conclusion that running economy is impaired by increased flexibility. I could vouch for them. And in a British medical journal two Australian researchers found that stretching didn't do anything to prevent DOMS (delayed onset muscle soreness) or injury. And from their data they said that it would take about 23 years of stretching to prevent one injury!

Warm up stretches that I like to do are all active moving stretches. Like leg swings, side to side standing hamstring stretch, bent knee forward and backward stretch, calf stretch while moving the knee straight and locked to bent, standing circle core stretch rotating your upper body in a circle with your hips still to stretch your abdominals, lower back and oblique muscles and maybe some arm swings too to get the shoulders ready. If you want to release muscle spindles (cramps) in your legs from running, the best way to do it is a deep tissue massage. This increases blood flow, releases the muscle spindle, and doesn't increase your flexibility. All of which are positive things. If you cannot afford a deep tissue massage, like me, get a foam roller and like Ludacris, 'Roll Out'. Yes, that's a bad joke, but it is still good advice. Hold the foam roller on the tight spots for a while and let them release. This is preferable, in my opinion, to an actual massage therapist. No matter how good he or she is, they cannot feel your pain tolerance, or know if they should push harder. You do because it's your body. If you learn how to foam roll decently, you will be better than a professional massage therapist at releasing your muscles. But don't tell them I said that. Do not roll over your joints and try to put as much weight as possible on the knots in your legs. There are plenty of websites that can help you out in this area.

Achilles Issues

I think about ever runner who has run over two years has had Achilles issues. I was sidelined for over two weeks right before Big Ten Cross Country Championships. This was VERY disheartening… I really wanted to run. And most runners I talk to develop problems with their Achilles at bad times during their season. I guess there's really never a good time to have a bad problem, but you know what I mean. I have tried many things to get a bad Achilles good again, and have found bent knee calf raises to be the most effective prevention. But sometimes if you get an abrupt tweak, even a good prevention weight program can be nullified. I have finally found a VERY effective, sure for an Achilles injury that works and allows the runner to keep running even at very high intensities. I developed this workout myself when I got one from a knot in my calf that made my Achilles hurt very badly for the next four days. It kept getting worse and I didn't want to take time off so I decided to try and single out the muscle and work it out, and to train through it without causing serious issues. It worked. I was doing 11.5 second 100-meter sprints two days after I started this exercise with no pain. Sounds like a miracle drug add on TV, but this is true. Here's my super sweet Achilles healing injury recovering strengthening move:

1. Stand on the bad leg on stairs so that your heel is hanging off, and your toes are on the stair.
2. Bend your knee until you feel the spot that your Achilles hurts the absolute worse. You may have to move you heel around a little, but make sure you find the magic spot of pain.
3. Once you have the painful spot, hold that position, keep your knee locked where it's at, and the rest of your body motionless and SLOWLY move your heel up.
4. It should only hurt for one or two inches of up and down movement, that's where you want to hang out during this exercise. You have to strengthen that spot, so the slower the better through the painful area.

5. You can do this exercise before you run, after you run, in the middle of a run if it starts acting up, or even at random points throughout the day. I advise all of the above.

6. Once your Achilles is all better and you can complete your season, give me a call and tell me I am a genius.

7. Ok fine… you don't have to do number 6.

The Warm Up

Warming up correctly is always a good way to prevent injuries. There are many different opinions on how to warm up the best for a race or workout. I think the typical warm up for a race or hard workout starts about an hour away from the race. They start out with a three-mile run at a pretty brisk pace, then do some static stretches for 10 to 15 minutes, and maybe some ballistic stretching too. Then they do some sprint drills, put spikes on, do a few strides, get to the line, maybe do some jumping or a couple more strides, and then run. Time to pick out the flaws in this typical mid-distance runner warm up and then you might be able to formulate a good warm up for yourself or your athletes.

We'll start with the normal warm-up run of about three miles at a decent pace. I have heard Kenyans like to start at a near crawl and then dip to sub five-minute mile pace on the last mile. I know in my college days and post collegiate days when I warmed up with other team members we always went pretty quickly. There was some sub six-minute warm-ups I was on that I really did not enjoy. Running at this pace for a warm-up can "warm up the muscles" indeed, but they also can deplete glycogen stores, fatigue the muscles for the race, and the muscles may even get cold from that part of the warm up with 40 minutes or more to go before race time; especially if the weather is colder. Sweating profusely from wearing warm-ups and running this long and fast is also a good way to lose heat faster and lose water for the race. For all of these reasons I think the best warm up is 45 minutes to race time, 2-miles or less at 7:30 mile pace or slower. This will not deplete glycogen stores, will not allow the nervous energy from the pending race to be spent on the warm-up, the slow pace will still get blood flow to the legs to recover them, clear the junk from them, activate the muscles you'll use in a race and not cause you to lose excessive water. Basically, I slow jog around for about 15 minutes to get back to my stuff with around 30 minutes until race time.

The next thing normal warmer-uppers do is static stretch for a while, then run. This elongates the muscles causing the runner to be less efficient and doesn't get them ready for the movements that they are about to do. For this reason I'll do mobility stretching at this time, which means I'm constantly moving through stretches. This will not elongate your muscles but will get them ready for the hardships of the race.

The next thing an average warm-up will entail is a series of sprint drills generally done for about 25 yards and sometimes they do it back too. I generally laugh at this one; it does help tighten up the muscles they just lengthened while stretching, but this is a power workout they are doing before a race. These movements can fatigue the muscles very fast and deplete the glycogen stores faster than a quick sprint. I do like to do maybe two or three of these in a row to get my muscles ready for the race, but not any more than that. I focus on these after workouts and races to increase my power, not before. My all time favorite sprint drill before a race is the quick leg drill. This is where you take one leg all the way through your turn over as fast as you can. It's just a speed exercise with no strength; it's not a power movement, and won't hurt you for the race, but it does get you ready for a quick turnover. I generally do a few of these drills right before strides with my spikes on.

The next thing an average runner will do is a series of strides. I've seen some pretty darn long strides in my days. This is good in the sense that it will warm up a cold runner from their run that ended 40 – 45 minutes ago, but a longer stride can deplete glycogen stores again. I keep on talking about glycogen stores because they're vital for runners that run under an hour... or over. But anyways, a gradual pick up reaching max speed for 3 to 4 steps and ending before 50 yards is plenty for a warm-up stride. This is the most important thing in the warm up. You're directly activating the muscles you're using with a higher stimulus than you'll use in the race, which if done too long, will hurt you. But if done just enough to rev up the system, you will warm-up all of your different muscle fibers from just those few strides. This means that the three mile tempo run some runners do to warm up can be equaled by just two to four short, gradual pace increase, fast paced strides near the race. I like to do around 5 short strides around 15-minutes prior to the race spaced out a little bit. I always like to do these in as near to race apparel as possible. If it's cold out, I'll take off my warm-ups to do a stride and then put them back on afterwards.

My basic warm-up for a race or hard track workout generally looks like this. Around 45 minutes from race time I'll run 2 miles very slow, focusing on relaxing and breathing. After that I'll use the restroom then do some ballistic stretching for around 5 – 10 minutes. I normally sit down for a little bit intermittently and relax; chatting with somebody close by or maybe thinking about race strategy throughout the warm-up as a filler for times when I don't want to do anything strenuous but don't want to start the next thing yet. I like to shake my legs to keep the muscles moving without directly stimulating them... it feels good. Then around 20 minutes I'll put my spikes on and do a few quick leg drills and jog around for a little bit in the spikes too. Then I'll start doing some gradual pick up strides in race attire around 15 minutes to race time. I like to try to focus on controlled breathing and relaxing at this point, since it is really the main thing I actually have control over in the race and I'm normally pretty nervous. Then I rock out... Game Time.

Lane 7

Mental Game: The 10%

"America loves a winner, and will not tolerate a loser. Americans play to win. That's why America has never lost a war, for the very thought of losing is hateful to an American." (General Patton) Americans as well as many other cultures are becoming more and more obsessed with winning. Winning is good, don't get me wrong, but it should be a result of striving for excellence, not the end all be all. Excellence does not mean being the best, but instead excelling to be your best. Excellence takes passion and drive to keep doing the little things to get your self better and better. Without passion you cannot be excellent. All this comes from you. Drive to be the best loses focus on yourself and is externally driven, which leads to a loss of control. Athletes and coaches who are competition driven and need the sense of control will do anything necessary to control the ability to beat everybody else; namely cheating. The competition bug has destroyed athletes and coaches alike. Research has found that focusing on your own performance and working with (not against) others will result in increased effort, intrinsic (internal) interest (passion), enjoyment of the sport, better performance, less boredom/conditioned inhibition, greater drive/ motivation/persistence and increased the seeking of more challenging activities (Duda et el, 1995). Conversely, studies indicate that focusing on competition promotes many unfavorable actions that dwindle motivation/drive; one of them being a decline in concentration. The best athletes focus on themselves and what they have to do, not on what others are doing or the situation around them.

This mentality will also promote un-sportsman like conduct, including purposely harming others, and cheating (Johnson 1981). This makes a good deal of sense because if all you care about is winning then you will do anything to achieve that goal. And like I said earlier, you do not want running to be a means to an end, do it for the pure love of the game!

Mihály Csíkszentmihályi (good luck trying to pronounce that name!) introduced a concept called 'Flow' or being 'in the zone'. This is defined as, "A harmonious experience in which the mind and body are working together effortlessly; the mental state of operation in which the person is fully immersed in what he or she is doing, characterized by a feeling of energized focus, full involvement, and success in the process of the activity." We have all experienced this in one thing or another. This is the athlete's dream to be able to tap into this every time they enter a chance to perform. Does it make sense to focus on beating other people to enter into this zone? No. But concentrating on what you have to do, seeing yourself do what you have to do, believing you can do it, focusing on relaxing your efforts instead of straining to accomplish a goal and letting yourself do it regardless of outside circumstances will take you to your happy place.

Legendary Brazilian Soccer Player Pelé said this about being 'in the zone', "I felt a strange calmness... a kind of euphoria. I felt I could run all day without tiring, that I could dribble through any of their team or all of them, that I could almost pass through them physically." Notice how all his focus is all on him and what he could do? It didn't seem to matter if he was playing against better players or worse players, in a championship game or backyard pick up game; he was amazing. He did not let the external environment ruin his internal drive for excellence. This should be your goal entering any competition:

~ *Focus on yourself* – This is the only thing you have control over, may as well concentrate on that. Gain control your physical self well, and you'll have a good grasp on your mental side as well.

~ *"Screw the details! Leave the little things for little people."* Bill Hast-
ings, friend – Do not get caught up in needing to have every little
thing to go perfectly before and during a race. I'll let you in on a
little secret, things will go wrong. Focus on getting the big things
you can control right like: Sleep, good diet, warm up, and most importantly, Proper Training. Don't worry about things you can't really control like: a delayed race, being bumped around, people in
the race, little things that annoy you before a race, what type of
competition it is, etc.

~*Get in the Zone* – Learn to concentrate on the things that will put
you in this harmonious state of mind and body.

If you can learn to perform at your best regardless of the outside
circumstances I guarantee you will win more than if you let the
outside circumstances dictate your drive. Like I said earlier, I truly
believe that your training is at least 90% or more going to dictate
how you do in a race, but this is also very important. Do not get the
competition bug, get the excellence bug and try to do your best and
get better at everything you put your hand to!

"Improvement in running depends on continuous <u>self-discipline</u>
by the <u>athlete himself</u>, on acute observation of <u>his</u> reaction to races
and training, and above all on judgment, which <u>he</u> must learn for
<u>himself.</u>" – Roger Bannister

1. Brunel, P. (1999). *"Relationship between achievement goal orien-
    tations and perceived motivational climate on intrinsic motiva-
    tion."* Scandinavian Journal of Medicine and Science in
    Sports, 9, 365-374.
2. Deci, E. L., & Ryan, R. M. (2000). *"The "what" and "why" of
    goal pursuits: Human needs and the self-determination of beha-
    vior."* Psychological Inquiry, 11, 227-268a
3. Duda, J.L., Chi, L., Newton, M.L., Walling, M.D., and Catley,
    D. (1995). *"Task and ego orientation and intrinsic motivation in
    sport."* International Journal of Sport Psychology, 26, 40-63.
4. Johnson, D. W., G. Mariyama, R. Johnson, D. Nelson, and L.
    Skon. (1981) "*The Effects of Cooperative, Competitive and Indi-*

vidualistic Goal Structures on Achievement: A Meta-Analysis."
PSYCHOLOGICAL BULLETIN 89: 47-62.z

5. George S. Patton. Speech by General George S. Patton to soldiers going into battle for the first time. http://department.bloomu.edu/english/Patton.html

Lane 8

Diet:
Eating for Runners - Mind & Body

There are far too many different diets and ideas out there detailing what to eat and when to eat it. I have looked into some of the more popular ones and tried a few of them as well. I like to call myself a natural-born fatty. I easily gain fat weight very quickly if my diet is bad, no matter how much I'm running or working out. Because of this, researching proper diets and dieting tactics has developed into a passion of mine. Trying out different diets was a good way to see how my body responds, however, listening to smart people and learning from research articles proved to be the best. I have had good and bad things happen in the process but the outcome has been very successful for me, as I have come to a place where I can actually trust my diet.

I do not have a number of calories to count and reach, nor do I eat all organic foods, but I do have principles for my diet. Some are for weight loss and others are for recovery, or performance, or overall health. Some foods in the weight-loss category are included because it's key for me to be light while running around the track and I imagine most runners want to be as light as possible, considering the best mid- to long-distance runners appear almost dangerously skinny. But it's important to be mindful of a healthy weight; diet can easily cause a variety of eating disorders in obsessive compulsive-type runners.

For this reason, I think it's a great idea to face the issue head on. I have heard many dieticians suggest diets and guidelines that did not help what so ever. In my experience, they try to either help you see all food as equal or push for organic stuff. While well intended, I think the dietician world is far from the sports world; overall, dieticians just want people to be healthy. This is all well and good, but as athletes, we want to be teetering on a healthy life with the ability to do crazy physical feats that a normal person couldn't dream of doing.

It wasn't until I entered into the fitness world that I found the best dieting advice. I researched how body builders bulk and cut for competitions. Those processes provided a phenomenal wealth of optimal dieting information for any athlete, especially since it's so challenging for body builders to healthily lose more weight while at approximately 5% body fat. I don't think a dietician would recommend weight loss whatsoever, or even be willing to help. To stop mindlessly obsessing about it, I researched the details and formulated a basic outline that I follow because I truly believe in the following principles.

1. *Eat slow-release carbohydrates (SRC) throughout the week.* SRC foods are generally low on the Glycemic Index (GI) so they steady out your insulin production. SRC foods include oatmeal, whole-wheat breads and pastas, all-bran products, yams, beans, hummus, grapefruit, prunes, and nearly all vegetables. (Vegetables are the panacea for a bad diet) QRC's typically have a high volume with low calorie count. Even if they do not weigh much, volume is a strong mediator for satiety. When given low energy-dense foods, people at an all-you-can-eat buffet for a day have half the amount of calories, and eat 33% longer, compared to those given high energy-dense foods. (Duncan 1983)

   The opposite of QRC foods, quick-release carbohydrates (QRC) are high on the GI and tend to spike up your body's insulin levels, causing it crash soon thereafter. This makes you hungry sooner after eating. Insulin is a growth hormone that will cause you to gain weight or store food as fat if you do not use the energy created by it. QRC foods include sugary drinks, honey, and anything made from refined sugars and white flour like low-fiber bread and rice; basically almost anything refined and sweet. These foods do have their place, but if consumed in large quantities on a regular basis, insulin levels may remain high, which could decrease the muscles' insulin sensitivity.

Keeping your muscles' insulin sensitivity high will provide you with a much greater anabolic performance response to food consumption; your body will respond much better to taking a QRC like honey before a race and give you far more energy. The opposite of this, and obvious result of consuming too many QRC foods, is insulin resistance. This means your body does not absorb sugar as well and taking a sugary snack before a race will have little effect on your body, nor will it noticeably improve your energy levels. A diet high in QRC foods could also lead to diabetes, severe mood changes, adipose-tissue (fat) weight gain, and a high number of other health problems.

This is why carbohydrates have earned a bad reputation in the health and fitness world. However, carbs are the most important fuel for runners and non-runners alike. This is also why you want to eat SRC foods when you are not doing anything strenuous during the day. This will help you maintain a healthy weight, keep your muscles insulin sensitive, give you lasting energy throughout the day, diminish low-insulin level hunger pains, even out your mood, along with a number of other important health benefits. But you don't want to cut out the QRC foods out of your diet completely, which brings me to the next principle.

2. *Eat quick-release carbohydrates before and after workouts and races.* If you have been eating the SRC foods throughout the week, these will have more of an effect on you muscles and your sympathetic nervous system (SNS), which, essentially,

gets you ready for action. QRC foods will also increase your muscle glycogen faster than SRC foods. Your muscles' ability to use the sugar will not be hindered if you have been eating SRC all week. (I hope that made sense) I generally prefer to take shots of GU or honey before races.

After a race, it is also important to eat QRC foods because muscles deplete most or all of their glycogen stores, and runners generally have high amounts of Cortisol, and possibly, C-Reactive Protein in their systems; muscles are often torn up from the stresses of racing or working out hard. Eating QRC foods shoots up your insulin so your muscles start recovering and your muscles can absorb glycogen faster. The insulin production will also limit Cortisol production. Insulin is suppressed during exercise, so this will help. (Wilson, 2004) Having a quick-release protein will also help prevent further muscle catibolization and speed recovery as well. I like to have a sugary protein shake after workouts and runs; it helps me get ready for the next workout or race faster by speeding recovery.

3. *Stick with basic foods; don't change it up too much.* Variety causes one to eat more. (Ordman, 2005) Stay light on seasonings and different flavors. I try to keep my cupboards from having a variety of food most of the year; this helps avoid excess intake when not needed.

I've read that some people in other countries shop daily, buying only what they need for the day and don't even have a fridge! This is actually a pretty healthy way to eat. Too many Americans have way too much food hanging around the house, which causes them to keep on eating all day long. Some people believe snacking all day is an effective way to keep your metabolism up, but I think it's a good way to increase insulin insensitivity, gain weight, eat far too much, and always have to worry about food. Eating three or four times a day is fine.

4. *Solid foods are better than liquid.* Solid foods reduce your appetite most effectively (64%), as opposed to energy-containing drinks (0%) (Ordman, 2005).

5. *Get all your macros.* Healthy fats, easily digested protein, complex carbohydrates; absence of any one can cause unwanted cravings. The most important one is obviously carbohydrates. Protein is next, followed by the ugly, mean, unwanted stepchild who steals your lunch money: fat. It's necessary, but since your body can turn protein or carbohydrates into fat, you don't need a lot. The average American diet already includes far too much fat.

6. *Do not starve yourself.* This can cause binging and promote fat storage when you resume normal eating habits. Like I said before, three meals a day is fine, but don't miss one.

7. *Maintain healthy environment.* Your appetite is much greater for junk when you are constantly around boxes of donuts and pizza than containers of oatmeal or bags of freshly washed veggies. This relates to #4, above, as well.

8. *Eat polyunsaturated fats.* Fish, seafood, and grain products have the highest satiety ranking among fats. Omega-3 fatty acids also increase insulin sensitivity. Likewise, be careful with your consumption of monounsaturated fats: peanut oil, canola oil, and vegetable oils. They have a very low satiety ranking, which causes you to eat more than typically necessary.

   I know body builders who love to eat spoons of peanut butter to gain weight quicker. It is an effective bulking agent. But I also know very high mileage runners who consume peanut butter like it is going out of style and they remain super skinny. I remember hearing greyhounds run fast off of non-fatty foods, and huskies can cover a great distance at once and do much better on high-fat foods.

Since I run fast and not that long, I personally can't eat peanut butter too much, but I'll leave your decision on the matter up to you and your body.

9. *Keep a steady mind.* Depression, anger, worry, stress and just about every negative emotion can negatively impact your diet if left unchecked. This is probably why it's stereotypical for a healthy girl to grab a bucket of ice cream after she just broke up with her boyfriend. I don't know if this is totally true, but there does seem to be validity in it from asking thee opposite sex about the topic.

10. *RELAX!* You burn sugar mainly while awake, but only when you're body is most relaxed can it burn fat. Which means getting enough sleep, taking a bath or hoping in the Jacuzzi by yourself, deep breathing exercises, etc., all contribute. Relax in an area where you can totally relax and try not to have any distractions (other people, music with words, reading, TV, etc...) Learning to relax during the day could help you relax at night as well. There is no "magical fat burning zone", you normally only use glycogen stores while working out. EPOC determines how much fat one burns at complete rest to replenish stores. (Effectual post-exercise onset calorie consumption)

11. *Do not eat ANYTHING HEAVY 3 hours before bedtime.* And never snack at night. No sleep eating. Your muscles are less glycogen resistant in the morning. They are more glycogen resistant at night, which means you store more. I like to have oatmeal or a fibrous pancake in the morning to maintain level energy throughout the day, and veggies at night to curb hunger cravings and boredom eating. This is VERY important for proper weight loss. The most calories should be in the morning and afternoon to keep you energetic throughout the day. Unfortunately this is very un-American; we tend to skip breakfast, have a lite lunch, and

gorge at night. This will make you gain weight because you put your body into starvation mode and will store the food as fat at night when you should be using excess fat stores to replenish your glycogen stores.

12. *Eat a healthy fibrous high carb meal in the morning like oatmeal, high-fiber cereal, high grain pancakes, ect.* One of my favorite things to eat is my patented pancake in a bowl. I add pancake mix with some wheat germ to make it high in fiber in a bowl. Then I add water and stir till it's a good consistency and through it in the microwave for about 3 minutes. Then I have lite syrup or regular syrup based on the workout I have planned for the day. It's a perfect cheap delicious meal with very little preparation and clean up, that you can cater to what you're doing on that day for a workout. More sugar and pancake mix equals doing a workout. More wheat germ fiber with less sugar in the syrup equals lighter workout. Pancake equals delicious!!

13. *Caffeine = good before workouts.* It speeds blood flow, a vasodilator, increases alertness and readiness, and masks tiredness. I like it before workouts and races. BUT! It can upset stomach because of acid, and make you jittery and over nervous. Never take too much, test it with workouts before races. It can also suppress REM sleep and cause insomnia. Don't take it six to seven hours before sleep; caffeine's half-life is about six hours. Too much use can hurt Circadian Rhythms.

14. *Easy on acidic drinks.* Acidic bodies are more lethargic and store fat to buffer the acid. Pop AKA soda, coffee, alcohol, sugary drinks, caffeinated drinks and some black teas are good to go light on. While acid actually is a fuel source for your muscles, if you have too much in your system at rest it's almost like flooding the engine with gas while it's not

on. Very hard to start afterwards and not good for the engine.

15. *Not Much Alcohol.* A glass of red wine is actually a good thing for muscle relaxing, antioxidants, and calming effects. Anything more and most other types of alcohol can wreak havoc on a runner's body, immune system, sleep patterns, metabolism, mental functioning, and a host of other negative effects. If you can't stop at one glass, don't have any.

16. *Eat like a champion to be a champion!* :) Your diet is SUPER important as an athlete. Even if you're that skinny runner that brags about eating a large pizza every night washed down with three beers... I hate you. Just kidding, you rock. But seriously, if you have a great training program and get a good amount of sleep every night, you can still ruin your athletic carrier with a bad diet. Being in engulfed in the fitness world I know these are the three keys to health and in your case, performance: Exercise, Diet and Rest. If any one of those is out, it will negate the other two or at least seriously hinder them.

1. Duncan KH, Bacon JA, Weinsier RL. *"The effects of high and low energy density diets on satiety, energy intake, and eating time of obese and non-obese subjects."* Am J Clin Nutr 1983;37:763–7.
2. Dr. Roc Ordman, *"CHANGING YOUR BEHAVIOUR"* Beloit College 2005 http://www.beloit.edu/~nutritio/chngbehav.htm
3. Wilson, Ted. *"Beverages in nutrition and health"*, Publisher: Humana Press, Pub Date: c2004. pg 301

Vitamins: the good, the bad, and the illegal

In this portion, I'll review several of the vitamins and supplements I like and the reasons why I like them. You should talk to a doctor before taking high amounts of anything though. I heard that some doctors can take a blood sample and see what vitamins and nutrients you are deficient in and can tell you how much to take of which one. This information would be amazing for an athlete and if you can find/afford this treatment, I recommend it. But simple knowledge of some of the more important vitamins and minerals could help. Being an athlete, you will need more vitamins and minerals than the average bear. You use a high amount of vitamins and minerals from animalistic training sessions, loss of water, loss of fat, and recovery/adaptation. But make sure if you decide to take supplements that you periodically go off of them and see effects. Plus, it's a good thing to periodize supplements when taking. Here are a few and the reasons why I like them.

Calcium

Calcium is the most abundant mineral in our entire body. It regulates your heartbeat, blood pressure and water. It is also used in blood clotting, the maintenance and formation of bones and teeth, and the conduction of electrical impulses in the nervous system. And most importantly for you as a runner it makes your muscles work! If calcium levels are too low, nerve and muscle impairments can result. Skeletal muscles can spasm and the heart can beat abnormally; it can even cease functioning. You may also experience muscle cramps, nervousness, insomnia, elevated cholesterol levels, rheumatoid arthritis, brittle nails, aching joints, high blood pressure, tooth decay and irritability. It's hard to get too high with calcium because the gastrointestinal tract normally limits the amount of calcium absorbed. But still stick with healthy amounts and take a few weeks every now and then off of them.

Glutamine

Glutamine is a great amino acid for any athlete. There are numerous studies on the benefits of glutamine. Glutamine carries ammonia to the stomach to change it to urea in the liver or excretes it through the kidneys. Ammonia is a very deadly byproduct of amino acid break down, which happens when you workout. Approximately 50% of the ammonium or urea excreted in the urine is a result of glutamine. (1) Glutamine can also be used as a source of energy and is one of the most efficient non-carbohydrate substances to do so. It will also increase your total body glycogen storage, which is essential for a runner/athlete. (2) Glutamine also strengthens your immune system, mucosal growth, and lubrication which is vital for gut structure and productivity (3) And a great thing about glutamine is that they have extensively tested it and shown it to be very safe and effective even at ridiculously high levels.

Zinc

Zinc is a wonderful mineral. It promotes healing, cell production, tissue repair, and muscle growth. It works wonders for your immune system, helps prevent lactic acid build up, and can even aid in growth hormone and testosterone release. If you do not have enough you will lose muscle strength and endurance. Zinc can also be linked to a number of bodily functions like taste, sight, smell and even memory. This is a good vitamin to take at night.

Magnesium

Magnesium is a great mineral that helps the body relax, and even get deeper sleep. It releases cramps, aides in oxygen delivery to your muscle tissue, promotes muscle strength and endurance, and has also been proven to increase your ability to relax. Magnesium also activates enzymes necessary for the metabolism of carbohydrates and amino acids. These are all things that you want as a runner. This is a good vitamin to take with zinc at night.

Iron

This is one of my personal favorites because I am anemic. I remember getting tested for this and I had the lowest red blood cell count and hemoglobin in blood. Iron deficiency is the most common known form of nutritional deficiency. Symptoms include fatigue, irritability, pallor (reduce oxyhemoglobin in blood), pica (weird diet urges), weakness and brittle nails. (5) After I started taking iron supplements all of those symptoms went away. This could be a more dangerous supplement to take if you do not need to take it. Make sure that you should be taking this supplement before you start. Too much iron can be toxic; it mixes with peroxides in the blood to produce dangerous free radicals that can damage, DNA, protein, lipids, organs and even lead to death. So be careful with how much you're taking, and getting tested for anemia before starting is recommended. Also, getting tested after you have been on iron for a while is a good idea too. Vitamin A and C help iron absorption. B-12 helps with Anemia too.

Vitamin B

A Vitamin B-Complex is a great idea for an athlete to take. There are 8 B vitamins; B_1, B_2, B_3, B_5, B_6, B_7, B_9 and B_{12}. There are actually 23 other vitamins that were called a 'B' vitamin at one point in time, but these are the important ones. It aids in pretty much every step of energy production. It also helps with metabolic rate, healthy skin and muscle tone, immune and nervous system, cell growth and division, decrease stress and depression symptoms, and aid in cardiovascular functions. A deficiency in these guys will lead to a host of negative symptoms. It's better for your stomach to take this with food. Some of these B's have toxicities if taken in excess. Do not take too much B_6 (Pyridoxine), while proper amounts aids in a host of things, too much will cause nervous system problems like: disorientation, numbness of limbs, abnormal spinal cord sensations, impaired tendon reflexes, and degeneration of sensory fibers. The right amount will help all of those problems though. About 200mg a day should be your ceiling with this vitamin. That would be VERY difficult to hit through diet and normal supplementation though.

Hormones/steroids

This is what you use when you've given up thinking for yourself on how to improve your body naturally. They will increase your athletic performance. But there are a few drawbacks, and probably many more that are not even known yet. They will alter the way your body functions and may increase or decrease the amount of certain hormones naturally produced by your body. This is why you want to have these things done naturally and then your body will not be all out of whack. They could kill you. They will negatively alter your mood. Simply the knowledge that you had to cheat to get what you wanted will ruin everything you have work for emotionally. You will never really be able to fully enjoy the success you sought so desperately to achieve. It's illegal to use performance-enhancing drugs. Alter you training, not your body.

1. Susan Grable Shipley. *"Glutamine in total parenteral nutrition."* Nutrition Today, March-April 1996 v31 n2 p74(4)

2. Bowtell, J. L. et al, *"Effect of oral glutamine on whole body carbohydrate storage during recovery from exhaustive exercise"* Journal Applied Physiology 86: 1770-1777, Issue 6, June 1999

3. Chen K, et. al, *"Glutamine-supplemented parenteral nutrition improves gut mucosa integrity and function in endotoxemic rats."* JPEN J Parenter Enteral Nutrition. 1994 Mar-Apr; 18(2): 167-71.

4. Weingartmann, et. al, *"Safety and efficacy of increasing dosages of glycyl-glutamine for total parenteral nutrition in polytrauma patients."* Wien Klin Wochenschr, 108:683–688. 1996.

5. http://en.wikipedia.org/wiki/Iron_deficiency_%28medicine%29

Lane 9

Random Thoughts
& Ideas for Training

In this chapter I put a few of my thoughts and ideas that I sometimes use in training or think about. I just wanted to put a few of them down here and maybe they'll help some runner out down the road.

Racing and Pacing

There is no better practice than Racing and Pacing. I think a lot of runners are afraid to race a lot for fear of doing poorly, but if you want to succeed, prepare for failure! I'm not sure why coaches with teams do not use their athletes more to help out their other athletes. Pacing is the best way to do that for any mid to long distance race. Pacing is not to mentally taxing or physically, but in my mind it does help racing mentality and increase performance in the future. It also allows the athlete to give back to the sport a little, which is always good for the athlete; the more you give the more you get. It's a great extra workout for an athlete that has already raced or an athlete coming off of an injury and just wants to test out the racing legs real quick without a full effort.

Racing a lot is good for the workout itself. You can never perfectly create a race in a workout. If the runner can take the mental stress of racing a lot, I do feel that it is the best for increasing physical Performance. I have raced every season when I am not in peak shape and have run substantially slower than my Personal Records, but I know this will happen and am ok with it. But some people cannot take this mental stress of not performing your best all the time. For these people, training till you're in amazing shape may be the best bet.

One thing you should be careful of if you like to race a lot like myself is traveling. Traveling around the country or world is a fairly large stressor, and when added to racing can really take a lot out of you. I do love traveling around seeing the US and all the different track meets. But after a while when you are hoping onto a plane or off of a plane to race for a solid 6 months, it will get to you. I had to learn this lesson the hard way unfortunately for my 2009 season.

Workouts

Another one of my ideas for a potentially killer workout I have done a few times is a track workout with high intensity intervals followed by a tempo run of 20-30 minutes afterwards. My thinking for this workout is that the high intensity intervals will nearly completely diminish your glycogen stores, so the tempo run could teach your body to burn fat more efficiently at a quicker pace if there's no glycogen to use. It also could remove the excess free radicals from the high intensity workout you just did. But this is a VERY tiring workout, and shouldn't be done too often.

Another thought I had was doing a workout broken up throughout the day. Sometimes when you start a workout, you feel awful at the start and need to stop soon there after. Some coaches and experts will say, "do it tomorrow!" But I've had amazing success doing it later that day. I think the warm-up and few intervals you did revs up the system enough to come back and finish stronger later on in the day. This also may be why some runners, like myself, are really good at doubling on the same day. But I think that doing two high intensity workouts in the same day is far more beneficial than starting one and finishing it the next day. I think further field studies could be done on implementing this into your warm up. For instance, if you did two or three fast 30 second strides four to five hours before the race, this may be the best 'shake out run' you could do. I think Jeremy Wairner does something like this.

Running Shoe

Shoes are another thought I've had. Runners have waaaaay too much stability in their shoes that they walk around in and especially in their running shoes. I train in racing flats and Nike Free most of the time, even though I think the Free would be much better without so much heel padding. These shoes do keep your stability muscles working so when you put on spikes your calves do not become rocks and your feet don't develop plantar phashitis, Achilles tendonitis, or a stress fracture after a long track workout in spikes. I think most of the problems people complain about from doing track workouts could be solved with less stability in their shoes. I've read that before the modern shoe was made all the common running injuries were pretty much non-existent. You can also read about Native Tribes in the Sierra's running around for days kicking a ball through the mountains in SANDALs without getting any running injuries. This is another reason I have my runners run barefoot after every hard workout. Have to get back to their roots. I run barefoot too. Mostly I run barefoot on the track though... sometimes on cement, but only for a bit with no intensity. Great way to guarantee you run correctly would be to run barefoot on gavel! But you will most likely get cut, snap a tendon, or break a bone because the modern foot is so weak from the modern shoe. Grass and the track are probably a good start.

Base Building

I have heard that all coaches and runners advise developing a base before speed work. And generally do longer intervals before they do shorter ones. I think that this thinking is opposite. I think you should do shorter ones before you do longer ones; 58 second 400 meter intervals will feel a little less intense after doing 26 second 200-meter intervals instead of slow 800-meter repeats. Obviously, almost ALL coaches would disagree with this one, but I think speed should be what you build everything up from. It'll make slower longer runs seem a much easier. And I think that the quicker you can get your leg speed for very short intervals, the quicker your top end speed will be for every racing distance up. This is only a theory, I really have no idea if it's true or not. But from my observations of my own training, it seems possible.

If you are a first time runner or coaching one, this could be a very good way to develop good running form. Try running 'sprints' (fast paced for them) barefoot in the grass. Running form is usually better while running fast then while running slow. And this could be a good way to develop good form before cushioned, heeled heavy, stability running shoes ruin it. It will also make the slow longer runs seem a bit more relaxed and less stressful.

Training Analysis:
My Building Blocks

Well I love to look at the best training and base mine a little off of that. So I looked at two of the best, if not the best, mid-distance runners of all time. Sebastian Coe and Hichem El Geurrouj are in my opinion the best two mid-distance runners of all time. They had amazing form, great range in races, shocked the world with their feats of athletic ability and had great training. They had to have a great training program to do what they did. What I do here is just look at their training and talk about the things that I personally like, and the things that I don't like personally. Hopefully this will help you take a look at different training programs and decide what you like and don't like about them. Too many runners and coaches take one opinion or training scheme as gospel truth and this can kill you. Chew the meat and spit out the bones baby!! So let's start eating!

Building from the Greats

Training of Sebastian Coe: This is a random two-week period of Sebastian's training when he was younger. I'm sure he switched it up quite a bit being coached by his dad and having good communication with him throughout the day, week and years; but I still think it's good to see the intensity of his training.

Sunday A.M. 5 miles easy;
 P.M. 30 x 100m on slight hill at mile race pace

Monday 7 miles easy

Tuesday 7 x 800m a little under 2 minutes per interval with limited rest

Wednesday 11 miles easy

Thursday A.M. 1 x (400m + 300m + 200m + 150)
 P.M. 3 miles easy

Friday 4 x 1200m, 10 x 150m

Saturday A.M. 30 x 100m on slight hill.
 P.M.4 miles easy

Sunday 7 x 400m

Monday 7 miles easy

Tuesday A.M. 4 miles easy. 10 x 100m

Wednesday 3 miles easy

Thursday 1500m race in 3:50

Friday A.M. 4 miles easy
 P.M. 1 x (200m + 400m + 300m + 200m)

Saturday A.M. 4.5 miles easy.;
 P.M. 20 x 200m

Sunday 1 x (100m + 300m) + (2 x 400m)

Monday A.M. 5 miles easy.
        P.M. 5 miles easy.

Tuesday 5 miles easy.

Wednesday 3000m race in 8:14.2

   This is a very vague bout of training. It doesn't say the times of the intervals. Maybe it was a good thing to let the athlete decide what he felt like running for that day, which I do for myself quite frequently... ok, just about every day I do. But what I really liked about Coe's training was how individualized it was. He ran completely by himself almost all the time, and didn't even want to see his main rivals in any meet except at the Olympics. I think this is a good idea because it allows the athlete to run what their body should run that day. Not too much to put them in a hole, and not too little to diminish returns from the workout. I did not like the longer repeats he did, if they were on the track that is. But he was getting ready for a 3k, so he can be justified in that. I also didn't like the longer 11-mile run. I think he did this for pure recovery and didn't go very fast at all though. But I think you can get about as much active recovery from a 30 minute slow run as an 11 mile one. I think a couple of three to four mile slow recovery jogs is much better for recovery than one really long one. I liked how most of his repeats were 100 meters or 200 meters. This period doesn't show it as much, but I remember hearing that he was talking about how easy it was to run a 22 second 200 in practice the week before he got the 800-meter record. I think his 100-meter intervals really sharpened him up for the fast paced 200's, which got him ready for a slower paced 800-meter world record. Brilliant. I added some 100's in my training because of Coe's training, and it really does help your speed for all other intervals up. I think if you want to learn to run fast, 100 meters is the distance to build from. It does take a lot out of your muscles though, so give your self ample time to recover before the next workout if you run these all out. I dropped almost a second in my 200's after an intense 10 x 100-meter workout two days prior. And my legs were VERY sore. But I didn't feel great for a while after that workout, so be careful with this one. All that being said, if you run anything from the 40-yard dash to the ultra marathon, I think 100's can help your training program.

I also really like his weight training periods. Peter and Coe knew that in order to stay healthy and increase Coe's power per stride he had to get in the weight room, and he did this in the earlier part of his season. He did stop in racing season, but the program was based on using weights as an integral part of his training. I think you should keep your strength program all year and vary it up a bit here and there, but having it in any part of your seasons is better than nothing at all. I'm sure there are many other nuggets of gold a runner can take away from Peter's coaching and Sebastian's training, but these are the things I took away from it.

Training of Hichem El Guerrouj: I'm not exactly sure what he did specifically, but I found the following plan online and it's reputedly a log of his workout leading up to a 1500-meter race. Based on my own results and my analysis of Coe's work, the following reputed workout schedule for El Guerrouj seems quite reasonable for an elite middle distance runner. Maybe the times he hit are a bit quick for just about everybody else, but the idea behind his training is outstanding.

* () = what I added.

Day 1:
AM: 30 min of continuous running at 3:00-3:10/km (AE)
PM: 40 min of continuous running as recovery. (RR)

Day 2:
AM: 30 min easy running/ Active Rest (RR)
PM: 10 x 300 m in 35-36 seconds (Doesn't say what he took for rest, I assume it was as long as he wanted) (Pure Speed)

Day 3:
AM: 30 min of continuous running at 3:00-3:10/km (around 4:50 – 5 minute miles)
PM: 40 min of continuous running as recovery. (RR)

Day 4:
AM: 30 min easy running/ Active Rest (RR)
PM: 10 x 400m between 53-54 seconds with only 30 seconds recovery. (Speed Endurance)

Day 5:
AM: 30 min of continuous running at 3:00-3:10/km (AE)
PM: 40 min of continuous running as recovery. (RR)

Day 6:
AM: Rest
PM: Rest

Day 7:
AM: 30 min easy running/ Active Rest (RR)
PM: 10 x 300 m in 35-36 seconds or 6 x 500. (Pure Speed)

Day 8:
AM: 30 min of continuous running at 3:00-3:10/km (AE)
PM: 40 min of continuous running as recovery. (RR)

Day 9:
AM: 30 min easy running/ Active Rest (RR)
PM: 40 min of continuous running as recovery. (RR)

Day 10:
AM: 30 min easy running/ Active Rest (RR)
PM: 10 x 400m between 53-54 seconds with only 30 seconds recovery. (Speed Endurance)

Day 11:
AM: 30 min easy running/ Active Rest (RR)
PM: 40 min of continuous running as recovery. (RR)

Day 12:
AM: 30 min easy running/ Active Rest (RR)
PM: 30 min easy running/ Active Rest (RR)

Day 13:
AM: Rest
PM: Rest

Day 14:
Race: Adrian Paulen M. 1st_ 1500m 3:29.51

This training program influenced my own program more than any other. And, other than my own training program, this is my favorite training program of all time. I really took some good stuff away from this program. There aren't many details provided but I tend to be a holistic picture kind of guy anyway and I was able to gain some useful knowledge from this program and integrate key components into my own training program. I'll first go over the things that I really like about El Geurrouj's training system, then the things I don't like.

What I like:

I really like the way he balances active rest, aerobic endurance, speed/race pace endurance and speed. I completely agree with this type of balance and think that you will be able to do more of each with the right balance of each. I think it's good to have very different paces for these like he seems to have as well. If you're going to go for all out speed, go nuts! If you're working on aerobic endurance, keep it as quick as possible without losing form. If you're going for active rest, go really, really, ridiculously slow. Know what you're going for, and do it.

I really like that he only does race pace or faster on the track and does his aerobic work off of the track. The only time I want to get really tired from running on the track is when I am training really stinkin' fast. I think when runners train at longer distances at a slower pace on the track and make themselves tired they are conditioning themselves to get tired on the track at a slower than race pace tempo. This is not the mindset you want to foster for running on the track. I make myself pretty darn tired running slower than race pace hill fartleks, but that's all right for racing because it's absolutely nothing like a track. It's pretty easy to condition yourself into a bad pattern, don't condition yourself to get tired from slow paces on the track.

I also like his staple workouts. He seems to have a couple of workouts that he likes to do. I think this is a great way to train. I have my few workouts I like and I vary them up a little bit. Keeping to a set of staple workouts allows you to know where you are fitness wise. Decreasing the stress of the unknown is always a positive for runners. A little bit of change is good, which is why I change little things like rest and pace with my staples, but too much change can wear on an athlete.

I also like his two runs a day. This teaches your body to recover faster and gives you more quality work while letting your body adapt to higher stimulus. It also allows you to get more miles in without over stressing your body all at once. I have done upwards of four runs a day. For active rest days two or three short very slow runs seem to get my body recovered VERY fast.

I also like how he keeps his intense work during the week of races. I firmly believe that this keeps the athlete's body ready for the hardships of a race.

What I don't like:

Things I don't like about his training are few and far between. I really think he was a brilliant training mind, or his coach was. They were both geniuses in my book. And this is my book. So, here they are geniuses. But for me there are a few things that I had to revise because I am different. I did follow this training plan as close as possible as I ventured out on my own and did very well off of it. Here are the changes I made and the reasons I made them.

I do not like that he does not have hill work, longer slower intervals off of the track or weight room strength work at this point in the season. I do believe that you need a good amount of strength work during this part of your season to complement your speed on the track. Plus the weight room keeps you injury free from all the stresses of the track and racing. I also don't think it's good to go super fast for over 200 meters. I think these longer sessions of all out speed can take a huge toll on your legs for racing, and could make you burn out a little faster possibly.

My Old Training System
(Highly detailed excerpts from my online journal)

I think this training is good to see. It did get me in very good shape and I learned more about myself and running from doing this type of training. Everything in here I talk about in detail since it was the first time I ever wrote my own workout program. I was learning as I was going and kept a very good log of what I did and how I felt. Finding another elite athletes log with this much detail is nearly impossible. I try to keep a very similar training plan except I now add a hill workout in there and take a four to six day break when I'm really tired. Other than that, this is a GREAT training plan, and I ran faster than I have every done before in my life on it.

5-02-6
AM (11am): Ran 3 mile warm up with a good base pace. 4 x strides, sprint drills and static stretch.
-Workout: 4 x 400 with 60 seconds rest. (55, 57, 58, 59) 4 min rest
2 x 400 (58, 60) 4 min rest
4 x 200 (29, 28, 28, 27)
-Ran 3 miles keeping my heart rate at 60%, so really slow. I did this because if I went that slowly then I wouldn't deplete my glycogen stores but actually replenish them while using fat as energy. Could barely stand up after the workout, after the cool down felt GREAT!

-Did weights set 1 – 4 x 16 full squat with 90lbs. 10 seconds rest between intervals.

4 x 16 leg curl (45lb) + 4 x 16(65lb) leg extension

4 x 16 adductor + 4 x 16 abductor machine (120lb each)

4 x 20 lunge with 45lb bar

1 x 20 step up on Bench Press bench

3 x 100 sit-ups

3 x 50 back extension

1 x 100 calf raises with 90 lbs

1 x 50 bent knee calf-raise with 90 lbs.

1 x 50 toe raise with 45 lbs

-Swam 15 min. slow in the sun for fun

-Laid down 1 hr, never fell asleep.

PM (7pm): Ran 3 miles @ 55-60% max heart rate to take active rest. Felt very good after the run, yawned during the run.

-Stretched 30 minutes after run to decrease pain and avoid tightness. All stretches held for 45 seconds.

-Iced hamstrings for 20 minutes.

Feel pretty good, a very good lactic threshold training day at race pace or faster. Very confident in today's training

5-03-06

AM: Easy run of 45 min at 60%

Felt all right, little long, and my muscles were really tight. Then after that I had a massage for an hour. Very painful. But I think it helped me out a bunch. And it only costs me 40 dollars for an hour! And this masseur has worked on Olympic runners and he's here in my club!! Very cool. Still tight though.

-Stretched for a while in the Jacuzzi. Still tight.

PM: Ran with Brendan Mahoney 30 min pretty slow but not as slow as before. Felt good, had fun. Feeling much better!

5-4-06

AM: (7.5 miles)

Warm up three miles pretty quick to get heart rate and body temp up. Sprint drills, little static stretch, but mainly moving. Did pick up strides along the stretch I was doing repeats on.

Work out: Ran 5 x 300 {200-300 split}(26-40.4, 26-40.1, 26-40.1, 26-40.1, 25-40.1) My rest was full recovery, I based it on my heart rate and let it get down to less than 55% max. This took different amounts of time. Sometimes 3 minutes and sometimes 4:30.

After that I ran 5 x 200 (26, 25, 25, 25, 24). Full rest as above, took less time though

Then finished with 2 x 100 (12,12) same rest and less time very little time needed.

Cool down: 2 miles at 60% or less, felt pretty good, loosened up after pretty good.

- Lifted maintenance set of 1 x every leg muscle fast and until fatigue. With a lot of Abs and Back.

PM (3 miles)

Recovery run of 3 miles, moving at a good clip keeping heart rate at about 66%. Felt very recovered and good. Feel ready for tomorrow's Tempo!! Game Time.

5-5-06

AM (6 miles): Ran aerobic endurance workout. Kept my heart rate right under 80% of my Max so I could get all the benefits of increasing my aerobic capacity and Slow Twitch muscle fiber mitochondria, but not creating more lactate then I can flush out. Also not depleting my glycogen stores as much as I would have if I had gone over 80%. Ran for 41 min, about 6 miles or so. Didn't really worry about pace so much like I used to on threshold runs. Normally I would have picked a pace and run 5:20 miles or better for 3 or 4 miles, today I went a little over 6 min pace. But I would be depleting similar systems that I had used the day before and steadily burned out physically. I could tell that I had not used the same system as the day before. Just ran as smooth as possible and had my

Heart Rate Monitor start beeping as soon as I touched 80% so I'd back off a bit.

PM (3 miles)
- Same type of run, just shorter. This one actually hurt a little more since I had used the same system that day. But I think it still helped me a lot aerobically, the Kenyans do this a lot, except their 80% is a lot faster... working on it.

Stretched 30 min and rolled on the foam roller for a massage.

5-6-06

AM (7 Miles): Recovery run, kept heart rate at 60%, had to run real slow. Passed walkers, but got passed by runners. Yawned in the middle of the run a few times, but I had to keep the pace low. Ran for 1:20 and all I got was around 7 I think, so that tells ya how slow I actually went! It took a lot of self-control to let a larger women pass me on the trail, but I had to do what I had to do. This run was great, it made me tired, but at the same time I felt good.

PM (2 miles)
- This was another strictly recovery run, felt pretty good. Took me about 20 min to finish.
- Stretched and foam rolled for a long time, loosened my muscles up real nice!

5-7-06

PM (7 Miles) Warmed up 13 minutes at 70% MHR. Did no static stretching but only ballistic stretching and sprint drills. Did some pace strides because I really wanted to get these 400's on pace so I could get through more of them instead of busting out the first one and it hurting me for later.
- Workout: Ran 6 x 400 with 1-minute break. (58, 59, 59, 59, 60, 59) {5 min. active rest} 2 x 400 1-min break. (59, 57) {5 min active rest} 4 x 200 1 min break (27, 27, 27, 27). Very happy with today's workout. Kept wanting to quit every time I looked at the line where I started the intervals, but fought through my mental fatigue. After each interval set my HR was 220 Beats per minute, or 110% of max; so I know I

pushed it to the limits. Wish I could have sustained the 400's through 10 straight intervals under 60, but hopefully soon I will be in that shape!! I'm heading in the right direction at least! Still did 2.5 miles at sub 60 second pace! And I know I pushed myself to the max, because I measured my heart rate at the end of each set and it was a little over 220 each time! Boo-ya.

- Cool down of 21 minutes at dirt slow pace. Tried to keep heart rate around 60% but it didn't want to come down very much, probably because I had cranked it up so high in the intervals.

- Power Explosive exercises: I am not going to lift in the gym from here on out. All of my exercises will be for Power on each stride. This means explosive movements that mimic running in some way or at least train the muscles I use in running for more power. I did a high number of reps with as much force as possible.

  1. Jumping over a Hurdle on grass: 50 jumps both legs at a time as (All exercises done on grass)
  2. High Knee Jumps: 50 each leg, 100 total
  3. Karaoke high knee jumps: 25 each, leg 50 total
  4. Bounding: 22 each leg, 44 total
  5. Frog Hops: 25 total
  6. Straight leg shuffle: 100 each leg, 200 total
  7. Straight leg bound: 50 each leg, 100 total
  8. Single Leg High Knee forward up and sideways up: 50 each leg, 100 total
  9. V-ups for Abs: 50 total
  10. Back extension: 25 total, and couldn't do anymore… back sore!

PM (2 Miles)

Ran 2 miles at a little faster than normal slow pace, and my heart rate never went above 102! So I guess I'm recovering faster! Or my heart was too tired to beat fast tonight… who knows. Feel recovered.

Rolled on roller a little bit. Stretched too.

5-8-06

AM (2 miles)

Slow miles, pretty sore from the drills. Boy, you were right, lotta pain, all over pain. Those drills were tough!! But I think they'll be really good for me in the long run.

Midday 2

Ran in the middle of the day slow for an extra recovery blood flow to the sore legs. Still pain.

PM 3

More "junk miles to recover. More pain.

5-9-06

AM (5 miles)

Aerobic Endurance run. Kept the ol' ticker at around 79%, I read that's the most efficient spot to build Slow Twitch muscle mito-chondria without going anaerobic. Like I said earlier, the drills hurt me too much in the right areas, so I couldn't sprint. Coach told me that I might want to limit the amount of new things I'm adding to my regiment. He said I should limit the amount of sprint drills possibly to make sure it doesn't hurt the intervals. I agree, but I still feel like I need them for a more powerful stride.

PM (4 miles)

Another AE run, tried the new shoes I bought from Willie and they were great!

Rolled my legs out on the foam roller, still pretty tight, we'll see tomorrow.

5-10-06

AM (6 miles)

Warm up: 2.5 miles at 60-75% MHR, then some sprint drills, and moving stretches. Then put on the spikes for some strides and to make sure a repeat of yesterday wasn't going to happen. We were good.

- 5 x 300 (39.4, 40.14, 39.4, 39.4, 39.35) Rest varied, took as much time as needed to get down to 110 beats per minute or

55% MHR. First ones only took 3 minutes, then the 4th one took about 6:30, and after the last one it took 8 minutes! Guess that one hurt a lot.

- 2x 200 (25.6, 25.7) I was going to do 5, but it was taking to long to recover, and I was satisfied with the 300's, they were about a half a second faster than Thursdays!
- Cooled down at 62-64% MHR bare feet on the tack. Then shortened up the sprint/power drills to 50 yards of the ones I wanted to do, no hurdles.

1. Bounds – 16
2. High Knee Jump – 25
3. Straight leg shuffle – 60
4. Straight leg bound – 22
5. Fast Leg Cycle – 25 each leg
6. Weight room maintenance work: Shines, calves, Achilles, adductor abductor, lunges, step-ups, abs, back and hip flex work. Just one set and quick reps for more power.

PM (4 Miles)
Ran an Aerobic Threshold run at 77% mostly, felt pretty bad before the run, but it really relaxed a lot of my muscles! Also did a lot of rolling on the roller and Jacuzzi stretching as well.

5-11-06
AM (2.5 miles): Slow recovery run
PM (4.5 miles): Ran Aerobic Threshold pretty quick and comfy

5-12-06
AM (4.5 miles)
Ran an Aerobic Threshold. Not using the heart rate monitor anymore, don't like it. Just going by feel. Trying to go as fast as I can comfortably with light shoes. I think I'm around 5:30 pace, I should get quicker though, I feel like I'm getting in shape, but I know I'm not there yet.
PM (2.5 miles): Recovery. Went slow and relaxed at a VERY comfortable pace.

5-13-06

AM (9 miles)

Ran a time trial 1400. Wanted to go a mile, but Willie said I should cut it down, and if I feel good finish up, but if not, keep it at 1400. Sounded good, and I apparently felt awful after three laps so it's a good thing I stopped. Went through in 57.5, 1:58, 3:01, and finished with a 3:34. Felt really slow the second to last 200. I'm sure if somebody was there I would have been able to kick, I know because it didn't take too much out of me physically, but mentally it was grueling!

- I waited about 6-7 minutes then did a 400 in 59, and 3 x 200 in 27, :60 rest. Wanted to do 4 x 400, but that wasn't going to happen.
- Did more sprint drills for Power, all 50 yards. They felt a lot easier; think I'm going to go longer next time.
- Cooled down with a 30 min Aerobic Threshold run, I'm not sure what pace I was going, but I was flying. Felt really good; I think I like that cool down. Taxes your aerobic system after your anaerobic system is totally taxed.
- Did some lifting on my own, just some maintenance work to try and stay injury free. But I could use prayer!

PM (7 Miles)

Ran a longer one to get in a long day. Did it at a good click, but not too quick, I was still hurting from the earlier workout.

5-14-06

AM (6 miles)

Aerobic Endurance: ran comfortably quick for about six miles in a little over 30 min.

PM (4 miles)

Ran recovery run with Kevin, felt good; ran a little quicker than recovery pace, but it felt alright.

5-15-06

AM (9 miles)

Warmed up a little over two miles, and then did some sprint drills and active stretching. Willie came to the track right as I was about to start and gave me the new shoes I bought from him at a discount and he times me. Great spikes!

- Ran 4 x 400 (58, 58, 55{oops}, 58) (goal: 60) jogged around track and started 2nd set. 3 x 400 (58, 58, 59) jogged around track after a long drink… hurtin' for certain.
  4 x 200 (27, 28, 26, 26) (:60)
- Then I did a lot of sprint drills; bound, high knee leap, straight leg shuffle, straight leg bound, high knee in and out, quick leg, side leap, and single leg hop with a full cycle in the air (did only 12 each leg).
- Cooled down 30 minutes as fast as I could, started out kind of slow, but got pretty quick as I went. I love this cool down, all my glycogen stores are depleted from the intervals, and it forces my body to use fats as an energy source a lot better. Gets me in shape quicker!
- The work out was pretty good! I felt really good for the most part, and it was REALLY hot, and the wind was so strong on the home stretch my socks blew away! So the last 200 of every interval was really tough. I know I could have done a lot more if I didn't do that 55 second quarter. I thought I heard Willie call out 28.8 for the 200 split, but he said 28.0, and then I picked it up into the wind. Feel fitter though, and am recovering a lot better too.

PM (4 Miles)

Ran as recovery, pretty slow, felt better as the run went on.

5-16-06

AM (6 Miles)

AE – ran this really quick, took me a while to get going again, but once I got into it I was rollin'!

PM (5 Miles)

AE – Ran this quick from the start, not sure how fast I was going, but I was rockin' even faster than before!

Evening (2 Miles): RR – REALLY slow, just for pure recovery, hopefully it'll help! We'll see tomorrow, feeling alright right now though!

5-17-06

AM (10 Miles)

Warmed up 15 minutes because it was hot! Didn't need much. Then did some sprint drills and some ballistic stretching. Put on spikes and did some quicker sprint drills mixed with strides.

- 6 x 300 – 200 (43-28.3, 43.5-28.1, 43.2-28.8, 43.1-27.4, 42.8-27.9, 41.9-26.9) Rest after 300 was a 100-meter jog, after 200 a 200-meter jog. Non- stop until done.
- 4 x 200 (26.4, 26.9, 26.5, 25.9) 200-meter jog in between.
- Did 50-meter sprint drills for a bit. Very hot. Blister on left foot.
- Ran 21 minutes pretty fast, then jogged slow the rest. Took 9 minutes to feel smooth, and then I died at 21 minutes. Guess my aerobic system was taxed real well yesterday and couldn't rock it the whole 30 this time. Then I did a lot of maintenance stuff in the weight room after that. So the total workout started at 12:20, and hit the showers at 3, and I had it very cold and took a while to get me temp down. These workouts are killer but I think I'm getting in shape fast!

PM (3 Miles)

Did this REALLY slow, took about 30 minutes; didn't start to feel better until 22 minutes in. Killer workout.

5-18-06

AM (3.5 Mile)

Slow 30 minutes

    1.1 hour massage

    2.(3.5 miles) in 30 min running back home from massage

PM (5 Miles)

AE quick 5 Miles

5-19-06

AM (4 Miles)

AE quick 4 miles and 4 x100 meter strides race pace

PM (5 Miles)

RR slow recovery run, took a while.

5-20-06

AM (10 Miles)

1. Warm up 1 hour, 20 min run at average pace, sprint drills and active stretch.
2. 1200 in 3:02 … 10 minutes rest afterwards, and then 2x 400 (57, 57)
3. Sprint drills 50 yards, and then 30 minutes run at around 5:20 pace.
4. Lifted weights as maintenance.
5. Felt pretty tired, I think from Wednesday. I actually went slower for the 1200 than I did at the 1200 mark running the 1400 a week before. But this was by myself, in the wind, and I really had very little motivation to do it. Not to disappointed, chalk it up to experience.

PM (3 Miles)

AE, ran these miles as fast as I could for a VO2 max session and AE. Felt pretty good.

5-21-06

AM (13 miles)

Ran these pretty slow, took me about 1:55 to get done! I think that's the longest I've ever run before.

PM (4 Miles)

AE – Ran this pretty quick, and it felt pretty good

5-22-06

AM (7 Miles)

Speed/LRLT: Warmed up for about 20 minutes, and then started because Willie was there with some runners to time me. Felt the

pressure… j/k.
- Ran 10 x 200 (25.9, 26.3, 26.4, 26.4, 26.5, 26.1, 25.7, 25.5, 25.7, 25.1)
- Slow cool down this time, all I'm interested in is feeling good for Saturday this week. Did 50 yards of sprint drills and maintenance weights as well.

PM (3 Miles)

RR - 3 Miles not too slow but slow enough to keep the heart rate real low, and glycogen stores kept safe.

5-23-06

AM (5 Miles)

A little faster than an all out slow run, but I don't think quick enough to call an AE run.

PM (5 Miles): AE - ran as quick as I could, felt a little sluggish though

5-24-06

AM (4 Miles)

AE - ran a pretty quick for this, but for some reason still felt a little sluggish! Dag blast it!

PM (3 Miles)

RR – decided to run this pretty slow, needed to feel better than my last to AE days for my workout tomorrow.

5-25-06

AM (6 miles)

Pace Run for the Meet:
- Ran warm up of about 3 and strides and then pretty much got right into it will little other warm-up.
- Ran 600 in 1:29, 200 jog (50 seconds), then 2 x 400 (58, 58) with only 100 jog in-between (30-40 seconds), then ran 2 x 200 (28, 27) with 50 meter jog recovery (25 seconds)
- Did more power drills, but not as many, so I felt good for the meet coming up. Did two miles on the track bare foot to really get good recovery in for the meet coming up. Did

maintenance weights too but not many and not much weight.
- Really felt confident in this workout, it wasn't as hard as the other ones, but I feel like it really got in the right kind of intervals to lock in a pace you want to run, varying the distances like that.

PM (2 Miles)
RR- really slow two miles

5-26-06
AM (6 miles)
Ran this comfortably quick, not fast enough to call it an AE run though. Did it as up beat recovery
PM (3 Miles)
RR – Did this pretty slow to make sure I was fully recovered for the meet.

5-27-06
AM (3 Miles)
RR – Total recovery run, really slow.
PM (3 miles)
RR – just doing this to pump the blood to my legs.

5-28-06
RACE DAY!
Got there early to make sure everything was all right since this was the first meet I've ever done not being on a team. Everything checked out; had a track, lanes, no snipers and most importantly, toilet paper. Started my warm up with Patrick, my old training buddy on the Farm Team, since he was in my race. We did about three miles; it was nice and hot so I just wore the racing tights. Then I went to the track did some stretching, sitting around, sprint drills and a couple starts with spikes on. Then I took them off and sat around for a bit. Put them back on did some sprints and got to the line.

Race went SLOW!! Grrrr, I was hoping that they would go out a little quick since it was the fast heat so I sat on Patrick. But he only went out in a 62 high 63. Awful... simply awful. So I waited another 200 before I took it, I just didn't want to lead the whole thing in the wind from 400. Then it went pretty good from there, I went through at 2:03, then 3:02, then finished in a 3:46 for the win. That was the first time I've ever negative split a 1500, and I was leading in the wind! I was pretty excited about that for sure, plus I felt REALLY good the whole time, even with the wind! So that helps me have a lot more confidence in the training I'm doing now. Did a shuffle jog cool down on the track bare foot since I was doing the 800 in a bit. I had a Masters guy with me the whole time pumping me up and telling me over and over about how good I was, it was nice. Kind of like my own little after race cheerleader! Good man.

So the 800 was kind of weird. They changed the time SIX TIMES before we finally raced it at 2:15. We were all warmed up about 2 hours before the actual race went off. Most of the Farm Teamers just went back and did a little workout at the Stanford track because they were taking too long... ridiculous. But Kevin, Brandon and Mark all stayed! That's probably why those guys are a few of my favorites. So Kevin was the rabbit, and he FLEW out there in front. I was happy that I was able to be second for a little bit behind him until a Hungarian passed me at 150. Kevin went waaaaay too quick for my blood. I was right behind the Hungarian who was right behind him. Kev went out at 50 low and I was 51 low for the 400. That was my Personal Record (PR) in the open 400 meters. Needless to say the next 400 wasn't as good. I REALLY started to feel bad around 500, slowed way down for the next 200, and then managed to kick it in the last 100. Hit a 1:54 overall so I was happy I didn't completely die after going about 2-3 seconds too fast the first lap. After the race I was gulping air with my hands on my knees, got up to punch Kevin in the face and went back down. Ha! No, he's my boy, couldn't ever do that to him. :)

After that I did a lot of sprint drills, with most of them being around 100 meters. Afterward I went for a 30-minute tempo run to flush out the legs from the 800 and sprint drills. Then I gorged at a team BBQ after the race. Good training day, except for the gorge after the race. But it was nice being the official barbeque-r at the BBQ. Oooooo yeah!

5-29-06
AM (6 miles)
AE – (VO2 MAX workout) Thought I should do some VO2 work since I haven't really done a lot of it training on my own. This was probably one of coach Gags prime workout, except he did it on the track, and I hate doing anything slower than race pace on the track. So I ran 10 minute warm up pretty quick, then did 1 minute fast with 1:30 rest. My watch actually can be programmed to beep at each interval so I never had to look at the watch during the intervals! Boo-ya! This work out was good and it didn't hurt me at all for the next day. Well done.
PM (3 miles)
RR – Really slow on wood chips at Stanford. It was a nice change of scenery, but nobody was going as slow as I wanted to so I ran by myself.

5-30-06
AM (7 Miles)
LRLT (Speed/speed changing):
- Warmed up about 3 or so, did some stretching, sprints and lot of leg swings. My hamstring sort of hurt after Sunday so I was a little worried about doing speed today so I did a little longer warm-up run. Willie came out to time me, but I started without him.
- 4 x 100 straights (all 14) 100 jog, + 400 (29, 26) {55}, + 300 (29,13) {42}, + 300 (27.9, 13.2) {41.2}, + 200 (26.1), + 200 (25.9), + 400 (28.7, 26.1) {54.7} + 200 (25.6), and 4 x 100 Straights (13, 13, 14, 13)

- Had good rest on all of them, it varied, but basically I went when I thought I could do what I wrote on the paper or faster.

Did 50 yards of power drills bare foot on the football field. And a 20 min. barefoot jog on the track really slow. Felt good, was happy to get through it all with no hamstring pain. Did some weightlifting afterwards, a little more than maintenance because I wanted to strengthen my hamstring a little more with all the power stuff I've been doing.

PM (6 miles): AE run

5-31-06

AM (6 Miles)

AE – ran for about 34 minutes pretty quick, felt pretty good. Still not sure what pace these runs are at in all actuality. So we'll just say amazingly fast! WOOOO. Set headings towards dirt trails at amazing speed! Done. Breathing was good, I think the HR went up to 180 though, a little north of what I would've like, but it still felt like a comfortably fast pace.

PM (4 Miles): RR – Ran a little better than a trot, if I had to guess it'd be about 8 min pace or better.

6-01-06

AM (6 Miles)

LT/Race Pace/Race Preparation: This was the first workout I've done off of the team with some company running along with me. Steven decided to do the workout with me; he's a runner for a local college in the area. I did about a 3 mile warm-up and some sprint drills with a little stretching. 3 strides about 80 meters or so and we went into it. I lead everything because I wanted to make sure we hit the paces I was gunning for, but it was still nice to have him behind me on the track!

- Specs: 600 in 1:28 w/200 jog recovery (about a minute), 2 x 400 (58, 58) w/100 meter jog recovery (45 seconds), 2 x 200 in (28, 28) w/ 50 meter jog (25 seconds)

- Did all the normal 50 meters of power drills with Steven, and then we jogged barefoot on the track for 20 minutes. Did maintenance weights after we got back to the club.

PM (4 Miles)

RR – Ran pretty slow again, just to get the legs going and flush em out once again. My legs felt pretty good, the only thing that's a little weird is they were kind of Jell-O-e afterwards and during too. Weeeeird. Had difficulty sleeping at night too, not sure why. Down a few pounds, and didn't eat much that day... which could have had something to do with it.

6-2-06

AM (5 Miles)

RR I ran this about 6:30 pace I'd say, not too slow, but not fast enough to be breathing hard or anything, I figure two days out this won't hurt me at all to do a recovery run a little quicker than normal.

PM (4 Miles)

RR – Same thing; went a good clip to really flush out the legs, but still slow enough to recover.

6-3-06

AM (4.5 Miles)

RR – ran this in 3 little runs of 15 minutes, two at home, and one at a truck stop on the road down to Occidental.

PM (2.5 Miles)

RR – Ran this with Phil and Morgan, we were going pretty darn slow, and Morgan started pushing the pace, so Phil and I dropped back a little.

6-4-06

Jim Bush Invitational: 1500 in 3:41.21

AM (1 Mile)

RR - Shake out run of 10 minutes.

PM (6 Miles)

Warmed up only 17 minutes because it was really hot outside, about 98 or so. I did it at a good clip, but probably only at 6:30 pace or slower I'd say. Then I went back and did some sprint drills, did a little bouncing stretching, and some sittin' around doing nothing. They moved it back about 45 minutes from when they scheduled the race. Luckily it was hot out so I think that helped me stay warmed up. I did some strides with spikes on and then took them off and was barefoot for the rest of the warm-up on the football field. The ground felt pretty good because they had artificial turf with ground up tires as fake dirt. Felt great. Had to do some more sprint drills and strides after I found out there was going to be a long delay. For some reason I had a really big bubble in my stomach, like I had to burp or pass gas or something. I think it was the coffee I had. About 2 cups apparently did me in. No more coffee before races! Could not get it out for the life of me! I tried everything. Well, not everything because I never did get rid of it. Then they finally started the race, I was behind Sean Graham, a very good Farm Team guy, and he was behind the two rabbits we had for the race that were going to try and take us through at 57 and 1:55 or so for the 400 and 800. This was a load of malarkey. They went through at 60, which put me at about 61; then they noticeably picked it up and went through at 1:59, which put me at about 2:00. After that the rabbits left the track; Sean, and another guy that snuck in, lead for the next lap. I never heard the split for the 1200, but I made my move around the corner of the backstretch to take the lead. I felt really strong at that point and held the pace for the remainder of the race, coming through at 3:41.21 for the 'W'. Boom Baby! Then it took me a while to leave because everybody was talking to me and taking my picture; but I wasn't to upset. ;) Did a 3-mile cool down and drove all the way home to Los Gatos with Jim Sorenson right after the race. Luckily we were able to take showers at the hotel before we left. It was a long drive, but I was so excited about making it to nationals that I was wide eyed and smiling the whole way. Jim was asleep. So I drew a sharpie mustache on him. Ok fine I didn't, but it would've been amazing! He did get me later by putting my tea mug in my bed... I'll get my revenge!

Slept 5 hours woke up and went to work still on cloud nine and on adrenaline.

There were many good things about this training system. It got me very fast very quickly and allowed me to stay fresh because of all the extreme variation in my training. I really felt the different workouts I was doing were complementing each other and felt no need to rest or change. I continued this hard-core training all the way until Nationals June 22nd. It turns out that I really messed up by doing hard track workouts every other day from June 4th to June 20th. Then I started a short aggressive taper for Nationals. Up until then I had amazing workouts and thought I was going to blow everybody away at Nationals. But, as it turned out, while I was prepping my body to run very fast in the middle of my training program in the very end I lost all readiness. That brief taper the week of nationals caused my body to adapt to less volume, frequency and even intensity a little. This was a mistake. I got in a sit and kick Semi-finals heat at nationals which I felt should have been ideal for me, but due to that aggressive taper just prior to the Nationals I had lost a measure of fitness. If my body was ready for the last 600 meters that Bernard Legat ran in 1:21, I would have made it to the finals, of that I'm sure because it was ready before I went into that "do nothing" taper that did nothing but take away an edge. Lesson learned and training/tapering plan modified.

My Perfect Training System
Ok yeah, so it's not perfect and there are even things I've changed about it slightly since I started this book! But, like I said, there's always something you can do better in every area of your training, so keep striving for perfection! Here's what I did before the 3:56.00 mile at the Dempsy Indoor Invitational. I was training pretty hard for the couple of weeks before day one as well. I have not regularly kept a detailed log since the one I put in earlier when I first started coaching myself back in May 06. But I don't really vary it up too much, so the weeks leading up to Day 1 below were very similar to days 1 – 7.

Day 1:
AM: Hill   Repeats   (aerobic   endurance)   Leg   work   in   Gym
PM: Rest

Day 2:
AM: 15 – 20 min tempo (between 4:45 – 6 min pace depending on how I feel)
PM: 15 – 20 min tempo run + Upper body Navy Seal Workout

Day 3:
AM: 6 x (300 – 200) 43 – 40 second pace for 300's, 29 – 27 second pace for 200's. 100m jog after 300, 200m jog after 200. Leg Power drills afterwards
PM: Leg strength workout + 20 min recovery run.

Day 4:
AM: 15 – 20 min tempo (between 4:45 – 6 min pace depending on how I feel)
PM: 15 – 20 min tempo run + Upper body Navy Seal Workout

Day 5:
AM: 10   x   200   meters   26   –   24   second   pace.   Long   rest.
PM: Leg Strength work + 20 min of continuous running as recovery.

Day 6:
AM: Rest
PM: Rest

Day 7:
AM: 400 meter time trial: 50.5 seconds. (Los Gatos All-Comer Meet) 30 minute run afterwards.
PM: Rest

Day 8:
AM: Hill Repeats (aerobic endurance) Leg work in Gym
PM: Rest

Day 9:
AM: 25 min tempo @ 5:05 pace
PM: Rest

Day 10:
AM: 6 x (300 – 200) 43 – 40 second pace for 300's, 29 – 27 second pace for 200's. 100m jog after 300, 200m jog after 200. Leg Power drills afterwards + Leg strength workout. *Did this as early as possible to get a longer taper.
PM: 10 min recovery run. ***Start of Completely Shererious Taper***

Day 11:
AM: Active rest 20 min
PM: Active rest 10 min

Day 12:
AM: Active rest 20 min
PM: Active rest 10 min

Day 13:
AM: Active rest 20 min
PM: Active rest 10 min

Day 14:
AM: 800 time trial: 1:52, 400m time trial: 50.1, 2 x 400 all out, 3 minute rest (Los Gatos All-Comer Meet)
PM: Active rest 10 min

Day 15:
AM: Hill Repeats (aerobic endurance) Leg work in Gym
PM: Rest

Day 16:
AM: 15 – 20 min tempo + Upper body Navy Seal Workout
PM: 25 min tempo run

Day 17:
AM: 8 x 400 meters under 60 seconds. 1-min rest. Leg Power drills afterwards
PM: Leg strength workout + 20 min recovery run.

Day 18:
AM: 15 – 20 min tempo (between 4:45 – 6 min pace depending on how I feel)
PM: 15 – 20 min tempo run + Upper body Navy Seal Workout

Day 19:
AM: 10 x 200 meters 26 – 24 second pace, Long rest.
PM: Leg Strength work + 20 min of continuous running as recovery.

Day 20:
AM: Active Rest 10 min
PM: Active Rest 20 min

Day 21:
AM: University of Washington Race: 3:56.00 mile
PM: Rest

Since then, I have taken out the repeat 400's during competition periods. I am sure there are many other things I will tweak ever so slightly to continually improve my program. But that's the beautiful thing about life; you can keep changing and improving everything you do!

The wheel was invented a long time ago, and it keeps getting better and more efficient. That's what I encourage the readers of this book to do, don't believe there's only one way to train and one person's word as the final law of your training. Yes, you should listen to others for all they have to offer. Take what you think will benefit you and leave the rest. You don't want to reinvent the wheel, but taking the best and making it better is always advantageous.

This next section is all about my story up until the end of 2008. Hopefully you'll enjoy it and possibly learn some valuable life lessons from some of my mistakes. I did not write about my 2009 season, but basically never travel and race in big races too much in one season! I was so burnt out by the end of the season I almost hung up the spikes because I said yes to every big race I got into no matter when or where it was. I learned from it. Couldn't even do my taper properly because I was racing so much. But I will take what I've learned and apply it to the next season! But it will be different. Enjoy!

Section 2:

My Story

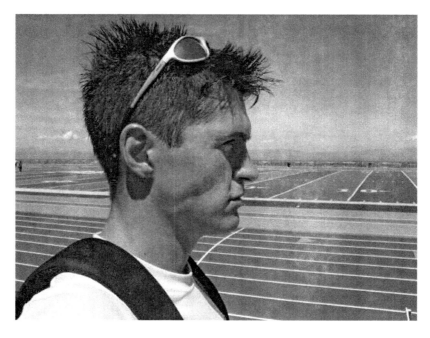

Everybody has a story; some are inspirational, others are educational. Certain stories are entertaining and fun to hear, while others are just boring. The tales your parents tell you 50 times with the same passion as if they were telling it to you for the first time, every time, fall into the latter category. This is not that story. This is a story about a man and his dog. Minus the dog.

Lane 1

High School: The Wonder Years

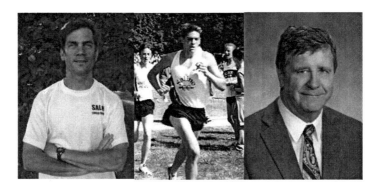

My High School coaches and me: (L) Tom Frederick (C) Me (R) Dave Medley

My story begins in high school, in the quaint little town of Saline (pronounced: Celine, as in Dion, the famous diva) in Michigan, just outside of Ann Arbor. I had been home schooled for the past three years of my life in a group of about eight other home schoolers. My class alone at this new school was about 400. Entering High School as a 195lb, 5' 9", home schooled, and somewhat overweight fresh-man, I wanted to be on a team to get to know people.

Everybody wants to be a part of something, so I decided to join the football team. Football players are cool, and I thought if I wanted to be cool, I should join the football team. I figured if I was part of the football team I would be invited to parties, all the high school girls would adore me and best of all I could be a star football player carried off of the field on everybody's shoulders after that game. The only problem was the guys on the team were not to accepting, girls didn't even look at me except to point and laugh and I hated hitting other people and/or getting hit, which made me a bad football player. Apparently you have to like running full speed head on into another guy (most likely bigger and stronger) who was also running full speed toward you with the intent of knocking you on your butt. I did not enjoy this behavior. I also found out, if you are scared to get hit, you're more likely to be the one flying through the air landing on your back with the other guy on top of you. I took a quite an assortment of punishment before I finally decided enough was enough.

I ended my illustrious football career sophomore year during practice. The offense needed to work on a play one random practice day, so I was on the dummy defense. I was the third-string defensive end, so it was my job to cover the outside and contain. The pulling right guard and the full back did not want me to accomplish my mission. They both hit me low pushing up to get leverage on me (that they didn't really need); as my feet came up in the air, all three of us came crashing down on my back. Luckily, neither of them got hurt; I, on the other hand, was not so lucky. As they got up laughing and smacking me on the helmet as if to say, "way to get owned", an overwhelming thought came to me: "AHHH HHHHHHHHHHH!!" I did not say this out loud, however, mainly because I had no air left in my lungs but also because I didn't want the team to think I was a pansy. But for days after, cringing every time I sat down, I decided my body could not take this sport anymore! Despite all the parties I wasn't going to and the girls I was terrified to make eye contact with, it wasn't worth it.

Ending football left me scared of being 'Fall Sport-less' so I joined the Cross Country Team my junior year. I remember talking to the coach and he said something along the lines of, "Well, try to run over the weekend. You missed most of summer practices but you do have to start running." I will never forget my first run for as long as I live. It was really hot and muggy. I think somebody put lead in my shoes; I stopped to check, four times... must've hid it very well. I stopped for pretty much everything on that run: I would retie my shoe laces, decided to stretch in the middle of my run, adjusted my socks once or twice, stretched some more and then stop to enjoy a scenic river next to the road. The only good thing that kept going through my mind was that I didn't have to run into a large angry fellow coming at me as hard as he could. This was my first three-mile run and I didn't think I was going to do well in this sport; I mean, I was a big ol' ex-lineman at the time anyways. After that demoralizing painful run I found it was easier to run with people. The next three miles I ran with the team, which wasn't that bad at all; it was surprisingly enjoyable to run alongside and chat with someone instead of getting knocked down.

It also helped that the guys on the team were really great guys and the coach was hilarious. The Boys Cross Country coach was Tom Fredrick and he had something funny and witty to say for just about every comment he received from us. He was also a pretty darn good physics teacher, I later discovered. Once, he almost hit me it the face with a bowling ball, but fortunately for my nose and his lesson, the law of diminishing returns held true. The guys on the team were all cool and fun to hang out with as well. Andrew Medley, Justin Russell and Andrew Ochs were three very inspirational team leaders a year ahead of me. Seeing how much it meant to them and how friendly and accepting they were as people, they helped me fall in love with the sport. This all made the switch from the football team to the Cross Country team all too easy; actually, crucial for me at this time.

Let me back up a sec and tell you why it was so crucial. Those first two years of high school were pretty much the worst two years of my life. Since I was home schooled all through middle school, I didn't know anybody except for one friend from kindergarten. That one friend would frequently ditch me whenever I made plans with him. My life was spent scared to decide where to sit in the lunch room, getting kicked off of the back of the bus by the cool kids, avoiding eye contact with everybody for fear they would make fun of me, getting rocked for a couple hours at football practice and coming home trying to forget the awful days by watching my brother play video games on the computer for hours on end. That was pretty much everyday of my freshmen through sophomore year of high school. I did get some sweet nicknames out of it though; like "Sherer the Queer" and "Chubs". Loved those ones... Okay, not so much, but to actually meet people who didn't make fun of me, who tried to get to know me, and pretty much accepted me for the first time in my high school life, was pure ecstasy. Because of their acceptance of me as a person, running became my life.

Another thing that helped me enjoy this sport was the results of my first time trial; I discovered I had a gift for running. We ran a 3 mile time trial up a long steep sidewalk, around the recreation center and back down the long sidewalk. I placed considerably well on the team after only two weeks of training running an 18:11 for my first race ever. I had never done so well or received that much praise from anything I did before in high school so I was easily hooked. I made more friends those few months than I had ever before in my life. Basically, runners rock.

I ended my first year of running cross-country with a Personal Record (PR) of 17:11 for 5K my junior year. Saline is always really good at Cross Country, and this year was no exception; so I didn't make the varsity team, but I did win some JV races. Since Cross Country was so much fun, I decided to do track too. I was blessed with amazing coaches in High School and my track coach was the best. Coach Dave Medley knew the sport of track and field very well and how to get his athletes to perform the best. He has a specialty with mid-distance runners learning from the likes of Peter and Sebastian Coe (I found out talking to him much later). He coached a 7:40 - 4 x 800 team 4 years after my team ran a 7:46 in 2000. He has always had very fast mid-distance runners because he knows what workouts make them fast. I have taken a great deal from his training style and I have not had more success from any other coach. He had me running 50-second 400-meter relay splits, and 1:57 - 800 meters splits the first year ever running. My second year ever running he got me to a 48.8 relay split in the 400, and a 1:51 split in the 4 x 800. He took me from being the practice dummy on the football team to 1st at States in the 4 x 800 (beating out Dathan Rizenhein's powerhouse team at Rockford), 2nd in the 4 x 400 and 3rd in the open 800 at the Michigan High School State Track Meet.

During my first year running, I will never forget the nerves of my first big race. My team and I made it to states in the 4 x 800 and the 4 x 400. It was a large scene, and this was the first time I really felt pressure to perform well. Every race before this I was somewhat of a 'nobody' beating people as the underdog. Now that I had made it on the varsity team, I had to come through for them on a seemingly big scale. I didn't notice it much on the ride over, but as soon as we were at the track, the nerves attacked. It was something I really hadn't experienced before, and I didn't know what to do with them. I really don't think I liked it that much at the time. I had some butterflies in my stomach and I sort of felt out of control, and wobbly. I mainly remember peeing more than usual. As weird as that sounds, it's true. Nerves seem to make me use the restroom constantly, and the extra water I drank on race day didn't help. It's also weird what nerves will make a runner think before a race. I calmed myself down by thinking that they were going to ask somebody else to run in my place. This obviously didn't happen; they came and got me to go warm up.

I warmed up with the team very quietly; they were saying the normal inspirational stuff teams say before big races while I was murmuring, "O crap o crap o crap o crap o crap o crap…" Unfortunately, my chosen mantra didn't seem to work, I couldn't even breathe deeply I was so nervous. After that, I really don't remember too much, probably because I became so focused on the race I forgot everything going on around me. To this day, my parents tell me stories from races that I don't remember at all, and this one was no exception. I remember part of the warm-up, the awards podium, and being very nervous all day, nothing else. I do remember that my split was a 1:57 for the 4 x 800, which was a two second lifetime best. For the 4 x 400, I remember very little as well. Even though I don't really remember the races, I will always remember the feelings I had before; they left a mark. I did start to like the nerves a bit more in big races later on, and they were never quite as intense as they were in that race. Now I have finally come to enjoy and embrace those feelings; however, I do try to control them a little better now. However, at that point in my running career, I had no idea how to do that.

Running at States was amazing; I ate up every minute of it and squeezed every last bit of excitement from each moment I could. But the race that will always stick out in my mind as the most memorable race of my life took place during my first year running. It was the last race of the regional qualifying race. The entire stadium lined the fence alongside the track to cheer for the last race, the mile relay, A.K.A, 4 by 4. We were currently second in the overall team standings for the meet. We had to beat Huron and I believe they had to get fourth or less. Andrew Ochs led us off with a fast first leg, but Chris Yee (my buddy who would run the 400 for University of Michigan later on) lead off for Huron in a much faster time (Andrew would also run for the University of Michigan in the 400 meter hurdles). I ran the second leg. I had to pass a couple of guys to catch up to the Huron runner, and I was right on his shoulder with 100 meters to go. Luckily, I got lost in the moment and felt little pain as the crowd's roar spurred me on. I passed him and was picking up speed going into the hand off. I handed off in the lead to Frisco Melendez who kept the lead as he handed it to Justin Russell to snatch the win. We figured out pretty quickly after that race that we had won the team title and we all rushed the field. It was the first time we had won Regionals in about 40 years or so. We were all jumping around in the middle of the infield, on top of the world.

This was all during my first year running; the next year was an even more fun than the first! I raced quite a bit, sometimes three meets a week and as much as four races per meet. I did enjoy racing frequently very much though; I accumulated a whole box of hardware! … That box is collecting dust in my parent's basement right now. I only remember being beaten twice that whole year and both were at the state meet. After my third place finish at States, I did have a chance to redeem myself at the Mid West Meet of Champions. Tommy Greenless, who had won the state meet, would also be running there.

The Midwest Meet of Champions was a fun meet where a bunch of senior athletes go, stay in dorms, and compete against other senior athletes from all the mid-western states. Jeremy Auer was also a great 800-meter runner from Michigan and was there to run the 4 x 800. He took me and some other athletes out to drive around the night before the meet. I never knew how much fun driving over a railroad track ramp at around 50mph was; but now, thanks to Jeremy, I do. He was also my roommate freshman year. His four-foot speakers in our ten-foot dorm room also made for a fairly deafening experience, but we definitely had a good time.

The meet itself was the next day, so we tried not to stay up too late chatting. We woke up to a blistering Ohio summer day. It was around 100 degrees with humidity; I don't know how hot the track surface was, but it was toasty. The other 800 meter runners and I got to watch a few of athletes get carted off the track because of the heat, which wasn't too encouraging. Luckily for me, I run very well in the heat. It's the cold that drives me bananas. The race went off and Tommy jumped to the lead. This was the first open 800 meters that year that I didn't lead through 400. (I'm a front-runner) I finally decided to kick the last 100 meters fast and won in a 1:52.6; close to a two second open 800 PR.

All this was quite the "runner's high" for me, I was a big fish in a small pond and man did it feel good. It's funny how the first two years of high school were the worst years of my entire life, and the next were the best two years up until that point, in my life. I definitely owe a good deal of my happiness at that time in my life to the sport of running. I like to say, "If you can learn to enjoy running your body into the ground and pushing yourself to the physical breaking point, imagine how fun the rest of your life will be."

Lane 2

College Years

A few weeks before I left for college I was hanging out with some of my close friends from cross-country. We were kind of dorks and had a heaps of fun doing very stupid things all of the time. We made some videos, dressed weird for dances, had DBZ parties (if you don't know what that is, I'm not going to tell you) ran through the woods with hatchets chopping down dead pine limbs pretending to be defeating armies of ninjas and other imaginary things I'm sure most people might consider weird.

Well, that one time we were hanging out before college we decided to make a ninja movie, so, of course we had to practice our bow fighting skills. I guess it's a good thing we practiced, because we were very bad apparently. I took a hard blow to the knee during this display of pure awesomeness. Unfortunately for me, you cannot run on a knee with a deep bone bruise, which I found out the next day. I was devastated. Running was my life, and now it was gone. My attitude quickly went south. I stopped hanging out with a most of my friends (probably because I was moping all the time), my girlfriend dumped me (probably for the same reason), and then I got shoved into college with nothing going for me. It was high school all over again.

I was amazed at how fast everything good that I had built on running left my life. Going in as a freshman that couldn't run was not easy. You kind of feel like you have to prove yourself, and all I could do was some fast intervals on the stationary bike. The guys on the team weren't as accepting as my high school teammates, probably because everybody was a High School State Champ in something. I was right back where I started, hero to zero.

My mom wanted me to talk to a guy named Phil Gillespie who led a group called Athlete In Action; a Christian Athlete Organization. I figured I'd give it a shot since nothing else was going for me. We chatted about everything I could think of, but mainly what I was going through at the moment. He related really well and pretty much told me that I was putting my water in "broken Cisterns". This was a Bible passage in the Old Testament Jeremiah 2:13 that says people were getting all their glory from things that will quickly go away, and not putting it in something that will never go away. Running was my broken cistern I decided.

From that point on I have not taken my worth, happiness, or who I am as a person from running. That made my coaches angry sometimes when I wasn't sulking after a bad race at all. They thought I "didn't really care" or something like that. I did, but I didn't control me anymore. This was one of the best lessons I have ever learned as an athlete. Whether you're a Christian or not you can learn from this. Once you let running be your everything, it will chew you up and spit you out and give you nothing but resentment. Call it what it is, a hobby, a great social network, an awesome way to stay fit, a fun way to compete and perform at your best in or anything other than your sole purpose in life, because it can go away in the blink of an eye. I eventually did get faster, and the team did finally accept me more when I did. But I knew the things that were more important to me, and that always kept me centered.

After I learned that life lesson, college was a blast! I had a VERY busy schedule at that time in my life. A few of the more heavily involved things I did was: joining Athletes In Action and eventually became the president of the group, was a part of Campus Crusade for Christ, (made some of the closest friends of my life from this group), joined The Living Rock Co-Op and eventually became the president, was part of the SAAC (Student Athlete Advisory Committee) and was a full time Student with three sports a year. I like to be busy, what can I say? Running was still a big passion in my life, but there were plenty of other groups and things for me to feel a part of, and meet amazing people in.

Running no longer held my social happiness and sole feelings of achievement in my life, and that was an important lesson to learn. I barely even hung out with most of the runners at MSU outside of all the practices and meets, which was every day and most weekends anyways. But all my closest friends and even the guys that stood in my wedding were all a part of Athletes In Action or Campus Crusade for Christ.

But despite all the clubs I was in and commitments I had, running continued to be a big commitment in my life through all of college years. Even though I was super busy, I still found time to hop on the stair stepper, get in the pool, go to the weight room before or after practice (unfortunately I did not lift with my legs at this point in my career so I got over training injuries every year in college) and spent many a hour in the training room patching up my injuries. Anything I could do to get better and run faster I did it.

I did like Cross Country very much, even though it was not my specialty, so I decided to compete in it for college. I did not get to participate in my first year of college, however, because of some bad high school choices. For some reason, some good high school friends and I thought it would be fun to spin around with bows, like star wars kid online, and act like a ninja warrior defeating hundreds of angry faced attackers. This did turn out to be quite enjoyable until it gave me a deep bone bruise that sidelined me for a few months with only a couple weeks before college started. I was healed and ready to go for indoors though.

In high school I was a 400-meter/800-meter guy. My first year of college indoor track, I had to pretty much wave good bye to my favorite race, which was the 800, and I became a miler. I had only run the mile maybe three times in high school, and now it was what they wanted me to do all the time. I wasn't ecstatic about that, but I was decent at it so I figured I'd give it my all. My first year I took seventh in the indoor Big Tens race, running a 4:09 mile. I scored. Yay. I was fairly happy about that, even though I really liked the

800. I was now the fastest miler on the team, so I started to like it a bit. I decided to focus on it more from that point on.

There is more prestige and history in the mile than most events, and that helped my decision as well. It was kind of a let down that they only had the 1500 in collegiate out door track and field, at this point in my life that race was sort of meaningless.

I opened up the out door season with a trip to Mt. SAC in California and it was good times all around. Since we were traveling with the Decathletes, we had to get there on a Tuesday even though we didn't have to race until Saturday night. This gave my room-mate, Jeff Mulder, and me way too much time to have fun, and we did. We took the mini-van around blaring the music trying to act gangsta' rollin' down the streets. This probably would have appeared comical to any onlooker seeing two skinny white guys from middle class, mid-west America rocking out to a hardcore rap song about prison life while driving in a mini van around Los Angeles. We had fun, and that's what mattered to us. After driving around town, we then proceeded to take the fun to our hotel room. After sitting in a hotel room for a week, we started to get fairly 'ancy' and had a hard time sitting still. Finally, after nearly five days of hotel room sitting, it was time to race.

I was feeling the pressure on this race. It was my first time traveling anywhere to race, and I think it added a little bit of pressure to the whole experience. I had just come off of an All American Indoor Performance and my coach had put me up in a nice hotel for a whole week in California for a single race late Saturday night. On race day Jeff and I didn't do much at all. I'm sort of ashamed to say that we actually watched *Home Alone 2*, two times that day before the meet. It's amazing what you'll do on race day to try and not think too much about the pending race.

I remember my coach told me one thing, don't lead. Good advice... should have taken it. After 200 meters I found myself in the lead, with Jeff right behind me in second place. I did relinquish my lead until 300 to go when almost the entire field passed me like a slow driver in the fast lane. I finished twelfth with a four minute 1500, five seconds slower than I had finished last time. Jeff didn't do very well either, he finished one place behind me; the coach yelled at both of us after the race, for a while. Little did I know that I would get yelled at for running slow by a different coach five years later in the same invitational.

Then I was pretty much burnt out for all of outdoor the rest of the year. I did manage to run a 3:52 – 1500 to close out the season, but I felt like I should have been able to run faster. I never felt dead legged running before I ran in college. The volume doubled for me, and my legs couldn't take the extra miles. I did know I needed more speed with less volume, but my futile talks with the coach only made him angry with me. Every time I talked training with coaches they got angry. I tried to put it in the form of "this is what I need to focus on more to keep running faster, the long stuff kills me". But I guess I could never quite put it the right cordial way, so my training didn't changed.

That summer, I decided to go out to Colorado with *Athletes In Action (AIA)*. They take part in a Summer Project, which is for all athletes from around the world, and it's put on every year. Athletes can either do the weeklong camp or a two-month long journey with AIA. I chose the journey. It was probably one of the most enjoyable summers of my life. I was living with about 40 other athletes who were really fun people and there was always something different to do.

One thing we all did was called the "special" which was a blast for an endurance athlete. Basically, we were put into random teams of about seven athletes, of all with different abilities. We then played all the other teams for 24 hours straight in different competitions, like: basketball, soccer, ultimate Frisbee (my favorite), swimming, volleyball, home run derby, tug of war, push-up contests, obstacle courses, touch football and other fun games. Going up against athletes that don't really run more than a few seconds per play gave me and the other runners a big advantage. My team had mainly endurance athletes, so we didn't lose a single game in any of the sports categories. However, we got smoked in the tug-o-war.

On top of all the fun competitions, they also gave us membership to a nice club to workout in and time to stay in shape. It was great training out there, and provided a much needed change of pace and scenery. I feel in love with the mountains out there that summer; made hill workouts a breeze. I came back very excited about running and about life.

I came back from Colorado to start my sophomore year in exceptional cross-country shape. I was having a pretty good Cross Country season, making the varsity squad, until an Achilles injury took me out right before the Big Ten Cross Country Championships. I had only made varsity one year in high school, but it had only been my second year ever running. I recently found a workout for the Achilles that helps it recover completely in only a few days; this information would have been useful at this time in my life. But since I didn't even know what Achilles tendonitis was at the time, I could only sit on my duff and mope around.

After my Achilles recovered and I was done moping around, I found momentary success in the 3K during my sophomore indoor season. Running a 7:59 to beat Ryan Shay was my shining moment my sophomore year. He was a great athlete, and to beat him was a big deal for me or really anybody. I did run a 4:03 in the mile that year too, winning the Meyo Mile at Notre Dame.

After these two back-to-back victories I thought I was the best runner in the universe, and would have no problem breaking the illusive four-minute barrier within the year. But shortly thereafter I started to burn out again just like my last outdoors season. I tried to hold on for nationals, but felt pretty flat by the time they came around. I held on to fifteenth place in the 3K at nationals that year, but I ran eleven seconds slower than my PR and didn't feel good at all during the race. Luckily, since there were so many foreigners in the race, I earned 'All American' honors, which was only given to the top eight Americans at nationals. However, I was still heading in the wrong direction.

I seemed to come around quick and burn out even quicker during college. I wanted to run some 4 x 400 meter and open 800 like I did in High School, but this was not going to happen anymore from this point on. I had learned to suck it up and say, "thank you sir may I have another!" the "another" being two mile repeats on the indoor track, a long fartlek on the river trail, a base run that turned into an all out tempo run, 1,000 meter repeats to get a 'bigger base' and the only speed work we did was strides before a workout. I missed that quick feeling I had in my strides before races in high school where it felt like I had to slow myself down so I didn't go to fast. I would have that feeling for a little bit at the beginning of the season, but would lose it quickly thereafter.

That summer, I decided to take a trip out to Yellowstone National-al Park to try and enjoy some longer training in a beautiful place I'd never been to before. I figured if I have to do high volume training, I should try to get a large base in over the summer. I also wanted to get out and do something different. Unfortunately, nobody else could make this month long camping trip with me, so I went by myself. It was a great change of pace out there training and camp-ing for a summer.

I met some cool runners out there from Furman University and ran with them a few times. But most of the time, I was by myself. I remember people telling me stories about mailmen running out there and getting attacked by bears. They advised people not to go places by themselves and not to run. I was doing both, and not in the populated area. Well, I'm no pansy sissy pants Mc Afraidian, but I do like to be prepared; so I got large canister of Bear Mace. It could shoot a forty-foot cloud of the strongest EPA allowed pepper spray, but it didn't work against a charging bear all the time I heard. However, I still went off running around by myself, but if a bird happened to take off near me I found myself half way up a tree.

This was also another much needed change of scenery that helped me physically and mentally. I biked upwards of forty miles a day, lifted every other day with my upper body and ran ninety to a hundred miles a week on trails. This got me really skinny by the time I arrived back home. I'm normally around 160ish, my peak racing weight is around 152 – 155, but I weighed around 145 from that trip. I found being super skinny on high mileage made the long stuff a bit more tolerable, but not staying injury free.

I moved up to top three on the Cross Country team after the first race of my junior year. I was always top five on the team from this point on. I had started to become more of a Cross Country runner. Despite spraining my ankle the week of Big Tens, I did have a really good race, running a 24:54 to get 28th overall. After that I had a bit of a hamstring problem with my left leg, same leg as the sprained ankle. This problem escalated after the Great Lakes Regional Cross Country race. I could barely even jog without hobbling after that first 10k race. My body apparently wasn't that good at that distance, and it was letting me know through my hamstring. To top that off, I sprained my ankle for the second time two days before nationals; this time I could barely walk on it. Unfortunately, with some added pressure from coach to be a team player, I reluctantly decided to run Nationals with my injured left leg.

I was sort of excited to run at nationals, this would be the first Cross Country Season that I would have finished with the team. The race opened up with a gradual uphill, turned into an even steeper downhill and then kind of rolled along in an alley the rest of the course. I was going to give it my all and I went out with the rolling mob of runners close to the lead pack in a 4:30 first mile. The only problem was that I had about 5.2 more miles to go, and even the .2 sucked after the first mile. My left ankle began to throb, and the hamstring on the same leg started to tighten and get more and more painful with every step. I couldn't relax because of the pain and consequently couldn't breathe either because my asthma flares up when I can't relax. It was a travis-sham-mockery.

The one memorable "highlight" of the race for me was running so far behind that I got the pity claps, "come on fella, you can finish!" Clap... Clap, Clap. People were crossing the course to try and see the race, which I was no longer a part of. One of them who tried to make it between me and the guy ahead did not notice how close I was, so I took him out. That was my last good effort I could muster up in that race, I used my football skills I had acquired in high school. I drove my shoulder down to get the leverage on him and knocked the guy over. Not very good sportsmen like behavior, but I was having a bad day and he wasn't a competitor, just an inconsiderate guy. I did finish the race to beat a single person out of two hundred and fifty one, my good friend and teammate, Jamie Johnson; who was apparently having a worse day. But we still joke about it to this very day, like a good friend should. At the moment we weren't too thrilled. Our team wasn't too happy either considering we were only one point out of last place. Winning by one point is remembered through the ages. Avoiding last place by a single point is generally not the inspirational story past on from generation to generation. To top feelings of humiliation from the race off, I got yelled at for running bad on the ride home. AND, I didn't even defend myself; I just took it like a man.

After that, I spent most of my free time with the trainer. They knew me very well in there. For a long time after that, my left ankle felt like memory foam. If you pushed hard on it you could see your fingers leaving a mark there for about 2 – 3 minutes after. As cool as it sounds, I was not too thrilled about it. I was also not too happy about my hamstring that was actually worse than my ankle. I do not remember exactly how long I was out of running after that, but I definitely did not run any indoor and outdoor track that year.

At this point in my career I was getting pretty frustrated. I did keep getting better, but I was always getting injured and burned out during Indoor Track and have nothing for Outdoor Track. I would always think back to my high school days when running a 1:51 felt like I was jogging during Outdoor Track.

I also had a rough time recovering in the cold Michigan winters. I had long since determined that after my freshmen year of college I decided that Michigan was too cold to run more than 5 minutes for most of the winter. This might have been why I always had a great outdoor season in High School; I didn't run too much in the freezing cold weather. I really wanted to move to a warmer college to train how I like all year long, but I never did. One would think that I would just get used to the weather, but it actually got worse every year. I dreaded the bitter cold weather more and every year. I even started to stop in the middle of runs and go in buildings during runs to warm my hands and toes; this took a long time.

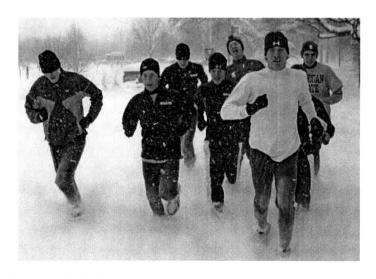

That's me in the back jumping up. Focusing more on the camera then the run.

My senior year of college I had a very good season in Cross Country. I was 42nd in Big Tens, and even did better in the Regional Cross Country Meet to finish 26th overall. However, this was not good enough to get me into nationals though, and our team was not very strong that year either. I did have a really good indoor season though, I ran a 14:02 5k, a race I was not a big fan of, but I did it. Then I ran another 7:59 3k, and a 4:01 mile to top it off. I even got sixth in the mile at Indoor Nationals, which was really cool because I was used to already being burnt out by this time in the season. That came shortly thereafter, though, and I had another dead legged outdoor season. I do remember I ran well at Ohio State University in the Jesse Owens Classic.

It was a beautiful night with very little wind, perfect conditions to run fast. I was in the 5k, hoping to qualify for Regionals; this was my last chance. I was kind of worried because I wasn't feeling great at all and I hadn't run well that outdoor season in any event. Tim Broe, a great Michigan runner, was in my race. He was just getting ready for the Olympic Trials later on that season, in which he won that year. It was a great race, paced well and smooth. Tim Broe was with us for the first mile or so, and then he took off. I tried to chase him, but could come to close. That race hurt real bad, I was completely by myself for a while in that race. I had to hold pace for a little over a mile by myself. I did think about stepping off the track more than once in that race, but I didn't. I managed to gut out a 14:15 5k, three seconds under the Regional Qualifying mark. This made all the pain I had during the race go away quickly there after.

Some of my close friends really wanted to go on a camping trip after finals. I thought long and hard about it for ten seconds and said, "Let's do it." This turned into a five-day camping trip over one of the wettest weekends in Michigan's history. We set up the campsite with four tents, numerous rope lights, a good speaker system in the middle under a picnic tent and a limitless supply of fresh mud. The main tent had an air mattress, electric heater, television, Sega game system, computer and tons of blankets. This was the girl's tent.

I was with the guys in the four-person pop up tent with five guys. Because of this no one could turn sideways for fear of spooning and we had to cross our arms because we all had really broad shoulders. This made for an interesting night of not much sleep. I did have Big Tens in a week, so this might not have been the best performance enhancing choices. But I am glad I did it. Big Tens was a sit and kick race in the 5k that year, but I was still dead legged like the race before and couldn't change gears with the rest of the field. The Regional Race went exactly the same way and I got the same place, 11th.

My Super Senior Year (5th year) I had my best Cross Country season. I finished 12th in Big Tens, 23rd at the Great Lakes Regional on a very hilly course, but was again fried for Nationals. We had a new coach for my last year at MSU and his coaching philosophy was about identical to the old coach's training. This year I had the worst indoor season of my entire career. I opened with an 8:20 – 3k on my favorite track and ended with the slowest Mile split of my life in the Distance Medley Relay at Big Tens. Outdoors was better, but still not great.

I did manage to run a lifetime best of 3:45.99 in the 1500-meter race in Arizona. I also ran a 14:04 - 5k at Hillsdale to get a meet record and make the regional cut. I always liked that track and their coach, Bill Lundberg; a nice fun guy who loves runners. This was also one of the first races my older brother came to watch me run, which made the occasion all the more exciting.

By the time I got to the Regional race in Indiana I was too burnt out to make it to Nationals. I'll remember that night for a long time. There was a brilliant lightening storm coming in with light winds. On my warm-up all I could think of was that this is could be officially my last collegiate race ever. I remember thinking, "what am I going to do after this?" It was a very surreal feeling warming up by myself with only my ambiguous thoughts and the distant lightning storm rolling in to think about. It was my amazingly fun college life coming to a close.

Because of the lightening storm, they decided to move the race to the next day. They moved all the athletes and fans to the indoor track to avoid the bad storm brewing outside. Nick Willis, who was there representing the rival Michigan Wolverines, and I knew each other from Athletes In Action so we chatted a bit and had a late dinner together. Nick said he didn't know what he was doing in a year from then but if I wanted a roommate, he mentioned it would be nice to train with me in Ann Arbor, MI. At that time I honestly thought he was just being friendly to a lower class runner, but it actually did work out! The race the next day did not. I just remember a whole lot of sucking and almost being happy to be done, I was tired.

I guess my college career was pretty good. I thought it was disappointing that I never made it to Outdoor Nationals once. I did make it to Cross Country National's three times and indoor nationals twice. But the really big letdown for me was I didn't get much better after my sophomore year, and in my favorite race, the 800, I only got worse. I guess I had big plans that really never got fulfilled for my running career in college; I felt like there was more potential in me then was being let out.

Lane 3

Post-Collegiate

After college, I really didn't know what I was going to do at that point in my life. All I knew was that I was terrified of having to move back in with the parents in order to figure out what I was going to do with my life. I saw that as failure because I thought it meant I couldn't make it on my own, and the thought scared me even though I love my parents to death.

I started thinking about joining elite running clubs to get my running career off of the ground. I still had a sneaking suspicion that I had more in the tank then I was showing and I figured that a club of amazing runners would really help me improve to my full potential. I wanted to get away from the norm, so I was looking at clubs far away. I definitely did not want to stick around Michigan State; didn't want to be the "scumni" that never leaves campus after he graduates.

I e-mailed a few of the elite mid-distance running clubs and the first one to get back to me, and the one I wanted to join the most, was the Nike Farm Team. I knew they were primarily a mid-distance training group, and were reportedly the best in the nation. I figured if I wanted to be the best, I had to join the best and do what they do. This was both exciting and scary for me, but I did it. I packed all my stuff up in my car and moved across the country to a place where I knew nobody and wasn't very familiar with any-thing: California.

I guess when you move away you realize how much you really liked all your friends and family. It was a rough first few months. Luckily Kevin Elliott was my roommate. He was voted most likely to be one of the coolest guys ever; he didn't let anybody down. This made the transition easier, until he went to Europe for a month a week after I arrived. That was a tough month.

I started meeting with some of the guys to do summer workouts, which did make the transition easier. They were all really cool guys, except for that one guy that nobody liked. But I didn't know who that was so it might have been me. Nooooo, they liked me, they feed me peeps (inside joke). But I really did like hanging out with the team.

What I didn't like was my first workout with them. I met some of the guys at a place called "Rancho" one summer day for a workout. There were only five guys that could make it so we were all in one group. Jonathan Riley, Chris Estwanik, Jason Jabut, Evan Fox and I did 5 x 7-minute hill repeats. I almost stayed with them for the entire first one. I was so happy. On the second one, I was determined to stay with the group. They were flying, but I was training hard and thought I could stay with them. I hit the wall somewhere around 2 minutes of that second repeat, and it was a two foot thick, well laid, pure brick wall of pain. On the long failure stricken jog back to the car, to add insult to injury, I had to push it kind of hard to fend off a high school girl running me down. I think I held her off, or I stopped for water and let her go by.

To be honest, most of my workouts didn't go too much better after that workout. It was all similar stuff to what I had been doing in college, but this time I wasn't in the lead pack. I was getting smoked in the back with Patrick Sulliven, my training partner. It was nice to have somebody else to complain to about getting smoked in every workout.

The first five months in California were awful. I was always tired and dead legged, just like in college but worse! I remember one night after a hard long workout my whole body was throbbing. It was pulsating with my heart rate, which was holding steady at about 70 BPM. My heart rate is normally around 32 - 38 BPM even after walking around. I was really hoping I'd adapt to the training, get stronger and be a good racer because that's what I did best. In college I was used to running much better in races while having not so great workouts. But still, based on my pathetic workouts, I was going to have to pull a Lazarus (bring my running back from the dead) for my first post collegiate indoor season, but I was still confident.

My indoor season rolled around and I was excited. Finally, I was done killing myself in workouts and could race competitively in the season that I typically do the best in. I decided to run a mile for the first time back at it. I went to Washington University to run in the Husky Invite. I really like the track in there; it felt fast, unfortunately I did not. I stepped to the line and ran my heart out and dropped a 4:15 mile. I didn't really turn any heads in the track world posting that kind of time. It was 6 seconds slower than my worst time in college. The pace was just a shock to my system since we didn't really do any speed work or pace workouts. But being the optimist that I am I figured I would give it another go in the 3K, since I had some success in that race in college. So in two weeks we went up to U of W again and I sucked again. Running a blazing 8:45 - 3k... needless to say I didn't do the Usain Bolt double fist pump + point when I crossed the line.

Now I really had to dig down deep and hold onto my optimistic attitude that things would get better, just keep trying and you'll get some PR's (Personal Records) in Outdoor Track. But I still had some lingering thoughts in the back of my head that said, "YOU SUCK! QUIT!!" Ok, so maybe they didn't say exactly that, but I was still pretty frustrated with my running career. I had always said when the year comes when I don't get faster in something, then that's the year I quit. I am reminded of the 'despair' poster that has a kitten hanging on by a single claw and captions, "Sometimes when you keep hanging on, you just look like an idiot." I wasn't getting faster and it wasn't looking good.

One of the best things that happened to my running career was becoming a personal trainer at Los Gatos Athletic Club. That was the job that Kevin got me when I moved out here. I started learning all about muscles, how they worked, things you could work on to stay injury free, increasing strength, finding weak muscles and everything else that has to do with working out. It became one of my obsessions. As soon as I get passionate about anything I learn everything there is to know about it and then start to make my own theories about it. I started reading research articles and learning as much as I could about everything. The best diet, proper sleep and why, different vitamins, periodization with different kinds of working out, different types of workouts and when you should do them; I had become a regular gym rat. The club had emphasized a new program called, "Purposeful Training".

This was a new way to workout that was based mainly on the client's heart rate. It said the best way to increase VO2 Max and reverse biological aging was to spike your heart rate and then bring it down as quickly as possible. It also emphasized limiting your workouts to under an hour, because you dig into a huge cortisol hole if you go over an hour. Weather this was a clever marketing scheme or not, I was inspired. Mainly because I hate running over 50 minutes and I like higher intensity shorter duration workouts. This led me to read some of the workouts of the best runners in history: Roger Bannister, Hicham El Guerrouj, Sebastian Coe, and even Bob Kennedy. Mainly mid-distance runners, but I threw Bob in there to make sure. All this revived my passion for running, but also made me annoyed with the workouts I was doing.

I talked to the coach of the Farm Team about training with the 800 runners group instead of the 1500-meter group and I got yelled at... but reluctantly he agreed to let me do it. Unfortunately, the training did not change that much at all. I was still dead legged. A little better, but I still had bricks in my spikes. I did feel a little better but ran a tactically perfect race in great conditions and won the race in a 3:47... close to 2 seconds off my PR. But I think I had my season peak then because I started to get slower again.

My cousin and good friend Cameron came over for a week and we went down to Mt. SAC for the track meet down there. We had a blast, except for the running part. I got DL (Dead Last) in a 3:55, and that was with a kick. On the bright side I did go to Disneyland with Cam and Jim Sorenson, which rocked. "Steve Sherer, you just awed the world, making a 3:55 look like a fat kid trying to catch a school bus. What are you going to do now?!?! 'Why, I'm going to Disneyland!'" We got big hats and lollypops.

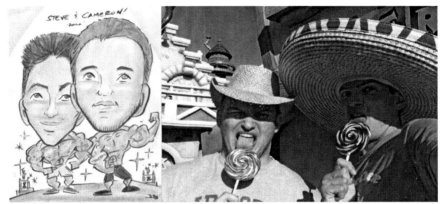

Apparently, this is how we roll.

I had a good time with Cam, but I was frustrated all over again with my running. And I got yelled at again for running poorly by the coach. Cam told me that he thought I was going to quit running after he came to visit me. That was sort of true; I was getting really sick of running slow. And reading all the things I was reading I wanted to try a different type of training but I couldn't because I knew the coach wouldn't let me train differently than the team. So that was frustrating on top of being frustrated.

The next race was up at Eugene Oregon, and it didn't go too much better. Actually it got worse, I sucked again. I ran a 4:01 - 1500. Then I got yelled at and kicked off of the team again. I started to get sad and have a little self-pity on my run after I got yelled at, but that quickly changed. I started to think that this could be my chance to train how I want to train, practice when I want to practice, run what race I want to run and not run when I think I've had enough. So instead of feeling sorry for myself I saw this as a great opportunity. Unfortunately, the coach said I could come back on the team, and I didn't have the cojones to say, "No, I think I would like to stay off the team". I had gotten yelled at too much, I was scared. But I also had agreed earlier to "rabbit" at the next race, so I figured I would at least stay on the team until I was done with my "rabbit" commitment for them. Then I sent in my resignation and started to coach myself.

Lane 4

Post-Team/Post-Coach Running

Ed Burke was one person who was proud of me for going off on my own. He had been an Olympic Hammer Thrower in the 1984 games and, more importantly at the time, was my boss. He was the owner of the Los Gatos Athletic Club (LGAC) where I was a personal trainer to a number of clients. Needless to say, I talked with him mainly about training ideas.

Another person I talked to a great deal about training was Willie Harmatz, a local shoe store owner and cross country and track coach in Los Gatos. He was a really nice guy who loved running and runners. He was my kind of guy. He definitely knew his stuff about running and really helped me get started on my own. He was the source of one of my favorite workouts that I use all the time in different variations: 6 x (300-200). You won't find that one in many books, but it's an amazing workout. He even came out and timed me a few times, which really helped being as it was the first time I'd had no coach or team. I still wrote all my workouts though. I wrote myself a very high intensity program going from May 5, 2006 to June 16, 2006 (see Section 2); I loved it.

I also used some workouts from El Guerrouj as well as his sequencing. I even used his strength workout and some of his power drills. I ran 2,000 to 4,000 meters total at goal-mile pace for pace workouts, or faster than 800 meter pace for speed workouts. I did a workout like this every other day. For the day in between I generally did one or two tempo runs of 30 minutes. And if there were days where I was a bit tired or thought I should just take an easy run, I'd run at eight to ten minute pace for pure recovery.

Since I was so motivated at this point in my life, I took a very extensive Captain's Log during this period. I recorded my pace for every interval, rest in between, and what strength and/or power exercises I did with sets, reps and weight. I logged about how many miles I ran that day, how I felt and even what I ate sometimes. I had never done that before or since that period in my life. Maybe someday I'll have the gumption to start up another extensive log of my training and life, but it does take a good deal of time to do and update on. I did put my log at the end of this book, so you can see some of the crazy workouts I did at this point in my life. I still do similar workouts now, but I have learned how to stay away from burning out now. For that reason, this training is good to know and use as the basis of your own program.

The reason I know this is a solid training program is because about a month after I started this type of training, the dead legs I had felt during previous training programs disappeared. I went to the Jim Bush Invitational in Southern California to run the 1500. This was the first time traveling completely by myself and paying for everything. I was a little nervous because my whole team was there to watch me, and I didn't want to waste all that time and money to run bad in front of my old team. Luckily, that didn't happen; I got a Life Time Best of 3:41.2 in the 1500 and had the season's fastest 1500 time on the Farm Team. A month before I was running a 3:59 – 1500's, feeling like crap the whole way, and only to finish the slowest on the team. This race was different. This race felt incredibly easy except for the last 100 meters, which sort of hurt a little, but the last 100 usually does. And to me, that's better than the last 1,100 meters feeling awful on top of running terribly slow. But this time, my time was about five seconds faster than I had ever run before and it also automatically qualified me for USA Outdoor Nationals! I had never even come close to making it to college Outdoor Nationals in any event ever! That race was definitely a break through race for me. Now I knew I was going to continue running competitively for a while.

Another thing that was cool about the race was that the whole Farm Team was there to watch and race against me. They say success is the best revenge, but I had nothing against them except for their training style. So pretty much, their training style owes my training style 20 dollars. And my colleges training style owes my training style 20 dollars as well. And somebody should just give me 20 dollars for running that fast. Just kidding. But seriously, I never saw my 20 dollars from anybody... Ok, so USATF did end up giving me a grant for a little more than 20 dollars, but they don't really have a training style. (Thank you USATF!) Ok, so if you're a serious minded individual at all times, please disregard this entire paragraph.

The next big race was Nationals in Indianapolis about two weeks later. I was really excited for this race, it was my big chance to show the world how brilliant my training system was and how fast I had gotten. Unfortunately, I got a little too excited. As my excitement went up, so did my training intensity. I did some amazing workout sequences, doing as many as four track workouts a week with the same high amount of high quality work. Everything revolved around rocking it at nationals; this was a mistake.

Once you give your life to a nasty slave master like track, it is like a bad boy/girl friend that sucks you dry and spits you out holding nothing but a note, "I'm just not ready right now, it's bad timing. It's not you; it's me. You're a great person and you deserve better... Blah, blah, BLAH!!" You get the picture. My track workouts did the same thing; once I gave it my all, it gave nothing back.

My fitness did improve for a couple weeks after my big race at the Jim Bush Invitational, but after that I started to get dead legged again. It wasn't nearly as bad as before though. I had very few workouts, so it was easy for me to see I was struggling when I had to use more effort to hit the same times. I knew something was wrong. I did feel all right after a few pure recovery days close to nationals though, but then things didn't work out in my favor. I got in a bad heat, and I'm not talking about the weather.

Nationals that year was definitely a learning experience for me. In my heat there was Bernard Lagat, Jason Lunn, and Said Ahmed to name a few. And unfortunately, when there's that amount of high quality runners in a race together, none of them wants the lead. We went through 800 meters in a crawling 2:10. This was the perfect situation for the experienced championship runners to just blaze a long kick. Lagat went around 1:20 for his last 600 meters to take the "W". I tried to go with him, so when he went, I tried to catch up, passing four runners on the turn as I went. This would have been great if the race was 1,400 meters, but they decided not to change it for me that day. After killing myself to catch Lagat, four guys ended up passing me on the home stretch. Only two guys, Legat and Lunn, made it out of my heat because of the slow start. And that was the bitter end to my season.

Despite that, I had a fun rest of the summer in 2006. I ran some All Comer meets at the Los Gatos High School Track that Willie put on. Also, I had an absolute blast with Kevin and the Farm Team guys the rest of the summer. Brandon Mahoney and I decided to jump off of a 65-foot-high cliff into freezing cold mountain water at Lake Tahoe. When I landed, my whole body went numb and tingly, partially because I landed wrong and partially because the water was freezing. It was a rush though, and I came to this conclusion about thrill seekers afterwards: the nervousness of looking at the edge, the threat of death, the thought of turning back but the over powering drive to say, "you did it", always outweighs the fear. And that's the rush people do stupid things to get. Some people need to jump out of planes, off of cliffs or bridges, fly down a mountain on skis, do a 360 on a snowboard or other extreme things just to get that "rush." I like to line up on that line putting my best against everybody else's to get that same rush. There are a number of people who can't take those kinds of nerves and will most likely hate racing for that very reason; but I've learned to love them. Especially when there's not freezing cold water coming at me near terminal velocity after the rush!

I had been talking with Nick Willis about living situations for the next year. Amazingly enough, he still wanted to live with me for the next year! So, I told him, "Twenty bucks and you got yourself a deal!" Okay, I didn't say that, but I definitely took his offer and moved in with him. I figured training and living with one of the best mid-distance runners in the world would be a good fit for me. He also lived in Ann Arbor, Michigan, my hometown and old stomping grounds. I was really excited to stomp Ann Arbor once again.

Lane 5

On the Road Again

On my way over to perform a perfect stomp, I made some stops. I visited some relatives in New Mexico, gambled with my grandparents and had a great time. After that, I went up to Colorado Springs to visit my cousin and best good friend Cam-o, or better known as, Cameron. He was playing his first Division I Air Force Football game, so I showed my support as I sat there and froze my butt off watching him. Apparently Colorado is cold at night, who knew? But coming out of boot camp for the first time and eating mainly crappy food, I think he was more passionate about getting to eat anything he wanted after the game than he was about playing the game. So I purchased front row tickets at McDonalds to watch the artist perform. It was all I had hoped it to be and more... like watching Michelangelo paint the Sistine Chapel. I also visited my relatives in New Mexico and my friend Mark Bojovic in Wisconsin. This made for a very long road trip around the US.

During this zigzag across the US I had everything that I owned shoved into my car. My Mazda was packed amazingly tight and riding super low on the tires the whole way. Not sure how it made it, but glad it did. When I pulled into the parking lot of our apartment it seemed like if I attempted to pull out a towel the car might blow up like corn in boiling oil. We had a bonus roommate named Mark Misch. 'Misch-man' as I called him and 'Chieftain' as Nick liked to call him. He was a top-notch citizen, and very down to earth. He could take more difficult situations than the average person and be all right with it. After a drunk driver going 60 plus

MPH smashed into him and his van full of athletes, trivial stuff doesn't matter as much anymore. It's also probably why he didn't mind living in a six by twelve-foot mudroom closet while Nick and I took the bedrooms.

Nick couldn't because he had too many clothes and shoes from Reebok and I couldn't because I just had too much useless stuff. I even managed to get a toilet bowl with a palm tree planted in it in my room to add to my 'completely useless stuff' list. I didn't tell anybody in the apartment, but just waited for them to notice a palm tree growing out of a toilet in my room. I don't think they appreciated it as much as I did... I thought it was funny. But anyways, back to Mark. He was one of the most passionate people about running and about runners. He loved the sport and the people in the sport. He had even been good friends with Nick's older brother, Steven Willis, before Nick cracked the scene.

One of my favorite Misch-man stories is the time I put a rubber chicken in his bed before he went to sleep. I expected him to come out and throw it at me that night, but I was wrong. The next morning he walked out with a confused look on his face and a rubber chicken in his hand. He said, "I woke up holding this in my arms... do you know anything about that?" Apparently, he didn't notice it at all when he went to bed. I couldn't have planned it better if I'd had George Clooney and eleven of his 'hommies' helping me. All in all, Mark was always a super nice guy that you could totally depend on for anything.

Another really cool roommate that I was blessed to have that year was John Scholl. He was a chill, down-to-earth guy as well. He ran for Arkansas so it was a running house indeed. He lived in the living room and was always fun to hang out with when he was there. Unfortunately, he was a busy guy and was rarely there. Actually, none of us really ever were home that much. I guess this might have been a good thing considering we had four post-collegiate guys in a two-bedroom apartment.

Moving in with Nick was a mixed blessing. I definitely learned a great deal from the experience. For starters, I've never seen anybody watch as many online races as him. I hope he watches his

Olympic silver medal performance as many times as he did other races because he definitely deserves it! From him, I learned that watching online races was a great way to learn racing strategy from the best racers out there, stride technique and so on.

However, once I moved in with Nick, I quickly found out that we have completely different training philosophies. He loves long distance hard runs and rarely goes under ten miles a run. I, on the other hand, rarely crack five miles per run. He likes long intervals around fields lasting eight to ten minutes, while I enjoy running on the track for 20 – 60 seconds. He'll go for an 18 mile run at sub 6-minute mile pace and I'll go for two runs of five miles for a long day. I did try to run with him for some of his workouts. We did some long hill repeats at the Arbs and I actually stayed with him, sort of. He stayed with me out of pity I think, but it was nice to run with someone again. I remember I went with him for one long run. It started out all right, brisk fall day running on mainly gravel roads. We quickly got lost and I started looking for moss on the trees. But he seemed confident so I stopped. After an hour my legs were becoming bricks, but I didn't want to complain. I complained after an hour and five minutes. But he did know the general direction and figured it out. I had not wanted to go over twelve miles; he dropped me off at sixteen. That was the last time I hopped on that bus... that crazy, fish-tailing-on-ice bus that threw me out the window at 100 mph only to hit a brick wall with my legs. Or at least that's how I felt.

It quickly became evident that our training styles just didn't mesh. He was a great guy, and I loved hanging out with him, but his training style just didn't work for me at all. It was almost like we went through a silent break-up, running wise. I slowly became more and more "busy" when he had to run. He began asking me less and less if I wanted to do a workout or go for a run. I started doing different workouts all together. Then Nick blew up and asked me why I didn't love his workouts anymore. I told him that it's not that his workouts are bad, it's just that they don't work for me. Then Nick started running with other runners and made fun of my workouts calling me a "glutton for speed". So I ran over his favorite pair of running shoes... repeatedly. Just kidding, I didn't... and Nick never blew up at all either. But it did have all the other signs of a classic break up. Misch-man was the 'other runners'; he liked longer runs since he was a marathoner; so it was a good match.

That winter, I decided to go to Africa with some good friends. I thought this would be nice for training because Michigan winters are awful and Africa is kind of nice all year. The only problem was that we were in a small mountain village in Swaziland with absolutely no flat ground. Every run I did was either straight up or straight down a mountain. And actually, tracks are not as prevalent in Africa as one might think from looking at how much they dominate at track in the Olympics. So I really couldn't train at all like I would have wanted to. It was a great trip and I made some good memories, but running wise, it pretty much ruined my indoor season for 2007.

I had one very memorable run in the mountains of Africa that winter. It was a cloudy day and this means that you're literally in a cloud on the mountains. I decided to run up the mountain, go figure. On my run up the mountain path I ran into a herd of cows. For the record, cows are EVERYWHERE in Africa. They are let loose, but not killed for food. They are viewed as a sign of wealth and you're not allowed to eat them. But I tell you what, if I was one of those kids you see on TV in those donation commercials, you would have to pan the camera over to the cow to find me. I would be the one cooking the wild cow and eating it to stay alive.

Okay, back to the story: cows, mountain path, and misty cloudy air. I stopped and looked at the ten plus cows in my path. All the cows have big ol' horns on their head, so while they may be scared of humans, commonly, humans like me are scared of them. If you took a horn to the face, it's game over man! I was scared... I never left the eyes of the lead cow. There was a dirt wall to the right of me with a ridge that was steep but walkable on top. I scurried up there, and I do mean scurry. It was very difficult, but I still held the gaze of the un-moving, un-blinking lead cow the whole time. I started walking forward, and then they started to move forward all together as well. As we passed, we were still looking at each other. Then I started to run, and they did too! It was really weird, I kind of wish somebody was there to see it, but that's why I'm writing it. As cool as that was, I left Africa and went back to Michigan.

I got back from Africa in the middle of a Michigan winter, and coming back at that time really made me miss running with the cows. It was so stinking cold! I have Raynaud's Syndrome so my extremities get REALLY cold, REALLY fast, and for a VERY long time. I put on four pairs of socks, long tights, pants, upper tights, 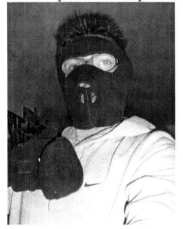 long sleeve shirt, jacket, two pair of socks on each hand, mittens over those, a snowboarding face mask, a wool hat and sometimes even ski goggles for runs outside. But I still would only make it five or ten minutes. This was no way to build a base or even train.

I've been much more bundled than this before

When I went to the indoor track at Michigan State during the open time I had to compete for a lane with ten older women that had to run side by side so they could chat... AND TAKE UP EVERY LANE! This really made indoor speed training sort of tricky, so I really could not train like I wanted to until April. This situation did not help my outdoor season at all and all the stress from trying to train in that cold weather was enough to almost burn me out psychologically! But I stuck to my training system and started to get fast again. I got in some races to run 3:45 or 1:49 by myself. Unfortunately, there were no rabbits in the Midwest and it was so windy, that fast times were hard to get being a post collegiate athlete living in the cold and windy Midwest.

I decided to fly out to the west coast to try and drop a few good times. At this point I wasn't even qualified for nationals yet and it was mid May, so I had to get in some faster races. I flew out to Eugene to get into a 'Road to Eugene' race that had a rabbit and some really good athletes. My good buddy Keverichio, also known as Kevin Elliot, and James Hatch lived right by the track so they let me stay with them. I got there early enough to do a track workout a couple days before the race. I was scared of the pollen and allergens in the air so I wanted to give it a test run before the race. I never raced well there before, the last time I ran a 4:00 minute 1500, so I was kind of gambling going there to get a qualifier.

The race went out alright; it's posted on www.flotrack.org if you want to see it. I felt pretty good throughout the whole race. I went out in a good pace; I was in the mid-pack hugging the rail like I like to do. I made a good move at around 500 to go to catch up to Matt Tegenkamp, but then my buddy Ryan McKenzie from my home towns neighboring country (Canada) had the best kick of the day. Although I didn't win I still got the A standard and a new PR of 3:41.0, so I was happy. What I wasn't happy about was that they spelled my last name wrong AGAIN in the results board... No "C" in Sherer!

After that, I flew down to Los Gatos to hang out with Jim Sorenson for a week and run the Jim Bush Invitational at Occidental College with him. Jim is a great guy, let me stay on his couch, watch his movies, eat his food, burn popcorn to the bottom of his favorite pot, and drive me around. I don't know how I have been blessed with so many really good friends, but I appreciate every one of them.

Jim and I have a few stories together too; from racing go-carts against each other at 60 mph, to getting attacked by raccoons camping in the redwoods. But my favorite Jim and Steve story is when we went to do a track workout at San Mateo. It was a great track with a beautiful overlook of the bay area. I forgot what workout he was doing, but I was doing my favorite 8 x 200 workout. At the beginning of the workout we were stretching together and I remember noticing a few plastic bottles clumped together at the end of the bench we were by. By the time I got done with my 200's, I was feeling pretty good and went to change into my shoes. What I found was Jim with a mountain of plastic bottles. Apparently, Jim has an addiction to recycling plastic bottles and he had collected every plastic bottle around the track like a champ! I was not going to be an enabler to his addiction so I started throwing the bottles back around the track until he learned. Okay FINE... I helped him carry the bottles back to his truck.

Then we flew down to Southern California to stay with his parents and run the Jim Bush Invitational in the morning. This time we didn't make it to Disneyland, but we had much better times in our races. I started off with an 800. I wasn't in the fast heat so we went though in a 54 second 400 which is kind of slow for fast times in an 800 meter race. I didn't want to go on the curve, but looking back, I probably should have. Instead, I went with 300 to go on the backstretch and ran a five second PR running a 1:47.7. My previous best open 800-meter time was in high school running a 1:52.6. My new PR qualified me for the 800 in the USA Outdoor Nationals, which was awesome. I was starting having a good outdoor season again, just like in high school! I decided to run the 1500 with Jim for a workout; it went out at a solid pace and then picked up pretty good at 300 to go. I finished second in a 3:42, but the real story was Jim who ran a 3:44! This was a new Masters World Record! How many people do you know well who have a World Record?! I only know one personally, Jim Sorenson. And I was in his race! It was all very cool. Good times, pun intended.

After that, I flew back home to Michigan to get ready for Nationals. All my workouts were feeling really good, and I really thought I was going to do well at nationals. However, Nationals turned out to be a learning experience for me.

I decided not to run the 800, which was a mistake on my part. I know that race; it's easy for me mentally. The 1500 can be psychologically destroying just sitting around waiting for it. There are just so many things that can happen that there's no way to be ready for everything. The 800's just a little easier for me to think about and race well. You would think that I would be better suited for a 1500 at championship races since I run a fast 800, but if you get knocked off focus for a second it's over. In most of those races they're going so fast that you have to focus on relaxing the whole time. If your body starts to tighten up it's hard to stop. And the first organ to go for me when I get into trouble is my lungs since I have sports induced Asthma. But if you're confident in the race, like I am in the 800, you're better at making yourself relax under high-pressure situations. I did not relax, and ran like a scared rabbit.

I shot out in the lead and tried to go out in a comfortably fast pace. I figured I'd just qualify for the finals by time from the gun; a little too bold of a move for where I was in my track career. I went out in a 55 second first lap, which was three seconds faster than I wanted to go out in. I pretty much lost the race there because I hesitated, freaked out about the time, and didn't relax the rest of the race. Everybody decided to pass me with 400 to go. I couldn't do anything about it; but in all honesty, I lost the race at 1450 meters to go. I really felt like this was an awful way to end the year and that I had so much more in me than that performance. So, I decided to go to Europe to race some more.

Lane 6

European Adventures

On my first flight to Europe, I decided I do not like long plane rides at all. They destroy you. I stepped off of the plane the first time in Africa to find that my feet and ankles were much thicker than normal. I named them 'kankles'. I figured out that wearing full tights does help your legs recover faster though. I think it keeps your legs from getting blood pooling in your legs with the decreased pressure for long periods of time and increases blood flow; so I wore full tights.

Mark Misch got me in touch with Murray Taylor a very nice "Kiwi". A kiwi is what New Zealanders call themselves. Who helped athletes get housing and into races over in Europe. I had never met the guy, never seen him, or even talked to him. We just swapped e-mails a couple of times and I headed over to Brussels, Belgium with Murray's number in my pocket, and that's it. When I got there, I found that neither of my suitcases made the flight with me. A girl I was sitting next to let me borrow her phone to call Murray. He said hop on the train and meet him in Leuven in about 45 minutes.

Well, I only then found out that my bags were missing. So I scurried to try to make a call from their pay phones (which SUCKS), but had little luck. I did manage to leave a message. But I finally filled out a missing bag report but it took forever. Half the airport was missing their bags that day. I finally made it to the train without contacting Murray at all, and got a ticket to Leuven. I made it there and failed to make a call to Murray. I thought I was going to pull an all-nighter in the train station in a foreign country all by myself. I wanted to rock in the corner in a ball and cry hard and long, but I stayed cool and maintained. Then, just when I was about to find the softest corner, I heard a weird British Australian type accent say, "Steve?" It was Murray! I felt like a boy who found his puppy. I still have no idea how he found me because he had no idea when I'd be there or too much of what I looked like. But I'm really glad he did.

I finally got to the dorm-ish type hostel we were staying at without my bags. I was exhausted but I had to find racing gear for the next day because I had my first race the next day. I borrowed Rob's (part American) Spikes and shorts, a Kiwi's (New Zealander) jersey, John's (a Canadian) shoes to warm up in. Luckily I did have my full tights to warm up in. I felt like I represented the world, it was a good feeling. Once I organized all of that stuff I showered and then laid down to prop my legs up for 15 minutes to get the junk out of them from the flight. Little did I know how much junk I would get out of my legs.

I woke up four hours later and it was dark out. My hands were above my head and my feet were up in the air; I was numb all over. I couldn't really move my legs or hands so I flopped over on my side and sat there for a bit trying to un-tingle my body; thinking to myself, "I'm sure glad nobodies trying to rob me right now, that would be embarrassing trying to fend him off." I slowly regained function of my limbs, but still had a headache. I fumbled around a bit for the lights, found them, brushed my teeth and went right to bed again feeling like a train wreck.

I woke up late the next morning and wondered down stairs wondering if everything that had happened the previous night was a dream or not. I had that slightly embarrassed feeling you get sometimes when waking up in unfamiliar territory. Downstairs I met up with Murray and another Kiwi and in their finest Kiwi Accent they said, "Morning Mate! Ready to go? We leave in 30 minutes." So I stole a couple pieces of bread from the cupboard real quick and ran right back up stairs to get ready. I threw my "world collage" of clothing together and went back downstairs and luckily, I made it to my first European Meet. Strangely enough, there were quite a few Americans there! I knew most of them, so it was fun to talk with them all, and meet some new people from around the world. I decided to pace the 1500 to open up out there, just so I could get rid of my plane legs. Also, getting paid for my efforts was a pretty good incentive as well. They gave me 100 Euros, which was "Meaty", as a New Zealander would say. They said "meaty" in every other sentence! I use to think Nick was weird for saying it, but apparently over there, it's like saying, "sweet". Anyways, I ran a 2:24 – 1000 meters to pace Chris Solinsky to his PR of 3:37. It felt pretty good, a little weird running in larger spikes, but I thought it'd be worse. The 800 I raced a few hours later was… in a word: bad. I decided to test myself in this race, so I went out with Jebreh Harris, a very talented 800-meter runner. He went out in a 24 second 200 and I was right there with him. He held on to win the race and I held on to absolutely nothing to get around third to last or something. I did learn not to go out as hard for the next one.

Racing over in Europe was a great experience and very fun; most of the fun came from hanging out with the other athletes. Rob Mandje and David Krummenacker were on my floor. Rob was hilarious, and David was just a cool dude that liked to play chess. There were also a bunch of athletes in the surrounding dorms, mainly from the US. Alan Webb was there among others. He even came down and sat near me in the lobby once and we chatted for 30 seconds! I appreciated it. I was the only other American to finish the mile race in which he smashed the American Record. I felt like crap and I was burnt out by then so I only ran a 4:07, but it was still pretty cool to be in the race… best seat in the house! When I came out to California again to coach high schoolers, they had all heard of me because I'd been in that race with Alan Webb! It was great to be known for running a 4:07 mile… oh well. It was still an honor to be in that race. I did a few other races over there; ran another 1:47 and a 3:43 or so. I was just burnt out again, I was getting frustrated. I kept on burning myself out and I couldn't figure out why. The question burned in my mind like a wood crate fire soaked in gasoline. I had to figure this out.

I decided to move back to California again. I just couldn't take the weather in Michigan, and 2008 being an Olympic year I had to put myself in the best position I could. I really didn't want to leave Michigan though. I have an awesome family and a good amount of close friends there. It was nice living near my parents; it was great visiting them as much as I wanted, and not just to steal some food and hop in the Jacuzzi... but it was a nice perk. I also got to work with my dad who works for Smith Barney and became a Marketing Associate there for a year. But both my parents have always supported me in everything I did, especially running; this made it almost harder moving away the second time than the first.

Lane 7

I Just Can't Wait to Get on The Road Again!

As soon as I got back from Europe I shoved everything in my little Mazda and took off for California again. The athletic club I used to work for said they would likely be able to sponsor me to be the spotlight of their personal training system. Unfortunately, the club did nothing to sponsor me and the guy that said the club would sponsor us, had gotten fired. They did give me a job, but they had no clientele after the old owner, Ed Burke, had sold the club. As a personal trainer, you need clients, so I had to find a job elsewhere. I ended up getting a job at Courtside and it worked out pretty well there. They have plenty of good machines and space to get a great workout in, which helps my training and business.

I also got in touch with Willie again and he asked me to coach the High school Cross Country team in Los Gatos. I love coaching, and I thought this was a perfect opportunity to get some real coaching experience. I coached with Karl Keska, a British 10K runner. He has quite the running resume to his name and he was self-coached as well so it was nice to talk to him about training. I also really enjoyed his sense of humor; it made going to the track a pleasure every day.

At this time, I had also been researching the phenomenon of 'burnout' online and in some books on training. I still had to learn how not to burn out. I also got interested in periodization and started looking into that too. I was always curious why runners

- 215 -

had such long periods for each and separated each system. To me, it was like separating your mashed potatoes with gravy, turkey, and corn; you can eat it separate and it's all right, but together it's what heaven must taste like. I also looked at lifters and how they periodized their weekly workouts; sometimes between muscle endurance workouts, hypertrophy, and power work. Some lifters only lifted one style for three weeks and then switched focus.

All this created a whole bunch of exciting new ideas in my head about what to do with my training for running. I knew that I didn't like long runs and high mileage, but perhaps it was all needed to keep from burning out before the longer season is done. I decided to try a four week periodized plan. I figured this would keep me from burning out if I switched my focus every four weeks, unlike having the same training program from March until late July. I figured I had some time to experiment and I wanted to try some-thing a little new, so I went for it. I wrote out an entire plan for the next three months with every day planned out, and then got started on it.

After a few weeks of this training, I quickly remembered why I really didn't like longer intervals and distance training. I was dead legged again. I figured you just had to deal with it for the base phase, so I pushed through it. Karl Keska said that it sounds good, but he likes to take a week break every three to four weeks of heavy training. I REALLY liked that idea. And the more I thought about it, the more I liked it. I even read that some of the weight lifters took a week down after about three weeks of serious lifting.

I began taking a week down in the middle of my phases, and it helped prevent mental and physical fatigue. However, I did notice that coming back from a down week, I felt really sluggish and heavy legged. But then I'd feel great the third and fourth workout in. I started to get into the last of the three cycles I had devised and decided to set up a race to find out how it worked. I asked Coach Willie to help me find some officials and I went to work trying to find the talent. I thought it'd be easy to find some track guys who were sick of training and itching to get in a race around mid November. Or maybe some cross country guys that ended their season early and wanted another race. But no dice. It was basically Tommy and me. I decided I wanted to run the 800, because I thought I could rock it. I think three people were in the race, maybe? Not sure, but I went through in a comfortable 51 and tried to hold on as long as I could completely by myself. It was a lonely backstretch I guess, because I finished in a 1:51. I really thought I had more than that in me, but it did help me see some flaws in my system. The meet worked out well for Tommy though. I paced him through 1000 meters and let him take the last lap hoping that he could get a better time. It was just him and me on the track again, but he still managed to get a lifetime best. I think that running program I made up might work well for him, only problem is that the system takes to dang long to get fast! I needed better.

Lane 8

New Day, New Way

I went back to the drawing board, not defeated but determined. I quickly thought of my new training system. It was a no-brainer really, revise the old system that worked, but fix the flaw; burnout. So that's what I did. I had three hard-speed endurance interval workouts, four to five tempo runs mixed in between the speed endurance interval workouts along with an unknown number of easy runs every week for two to three weeks. Then I would break for four to five days of easy running. I did this because it was long enough to recover mentally from the workouts. The typical two day break just isn't long enough to recover mentally because you're thinking about your workout in two days. I talked to Willie about it all and he said that it sounded good, but that I need some longer strength workouts in there somewhere. I agreed, but knew I couldn't do it on the track. I have a rule, no going slow on the track. Slow is anything above 60 seconds per lap pace. Obviously, I'm not going to do 800 or 1000 meter repeats at that pace, so I had to figure something out. One of Nick's workouts that I really enjoyed was a fartlek we did together on the trails. Typically it looked something like this:

1 minute hard, 1 minute easy
2 minutes hard, 1 minute easy
1 minute hard, 1 minute easy
3 minutes hard, 1 minute easy
Repeat 5 times

This kind of workout is a very long one for me, but I don't mind it that much because it's constant pace changing, which makes it go by quicker I think. Otherwise, 55 minutes of consistent pace would typically be harder for me personally. I did this workout a few times in Swaziland but I revised it so I would run up a mountain on the hard part, and jog down the mountain on the easy part. I really enjoyed that workout and since I had a mountain just down the street from me in California, it was done. This became my 'strength' workout. Even though I have a sneaking suspicion that the tempo runs help that area nearly as much.

Right as I was about to start my training, it was already time to go home for Thanksgiving. I love thanksgiving. Not because the day is really anything special in and of itself, but my family rocks! And it's always a blast to get them all together to laugh at the goofy things we all do. This year I decided to have a Turducken Party. This is a Chicken, stuffed in a Duck, stuffed in a Turkey all cooked together! Sounded like a brilliant idea to me so I threw a party over it. Cameron and I found out that it takes much more work than one might think. You have to de-bone all three birds! And on top of that, they're all freezing!! This is far from easy, but if it were easy, everybody would do it.

Throwing the Turducken Party was mainly an excuse to get all my friends together to have a good time and eat good food. I also invited a stunning woman named Kelsea Barondeau that I had been talking to online for a bit. I had only known her for less than a month, but she seemed like a breathtakingly amazing girl, so I had to ask. I was sort of surprised she said she would come, I tried to ask semi-jokingly in case she thought I was weird just for asking her. But she said yes. Since I asked her to come I thought the gentlemanly thing to do would be to buy a ticket for her to come out to Michigan and bless my Turducken Party with her presence.

We had a really fun weekend together full of friends, family and good times. I think there are very few more fun occasions than when cards are played at my house. Especially with the group of friends I had over that night; it was a riot. Then we decided to "watch" Transformers, but we talked through the entire movie. I guess it was just an excuse to stay up late and chat about life. We covered some good topics of which I will just say included a few 'hypothetical's'. It was great to talk about the 'what if's' before we decided to commit to anything, it really helps with the decision process.

The next day we had to get ready for the Turducken party! Cam came over and we started cooking some Turducken. As Will Ferrell likes to say, it was glorious!! The Best Turducken ever made, ever! After all my friends came over and ate, we proceeded to play a whole bunch of different games for most of the night. When everybody left, Kelsea and I decided to watch Pearl Harbor, but we just chatted and didn't even watch the second half. I'm a bit of a romantic at heart so I thought I could do better than just the movie. I recommend this next move to all guys who have great women in their lives. We skipped the second disc and went upstairs instead. I grabbed my laptop and took it with me outside. We went to my back porch to find a bright full moon with frost covering everything in a sparkling white coat. I played "You are the Love of my Life" by Michael W. Smith and we danced in the moonlight.

That capped off a perfect day and then we went to sleep. She took the nice bed in my old room, and I took the futon brick in the other room. The next day was nice, went to church with the parents, then to lunch. We had a couple of hours before she had to leave to the airport and go our separate ways, so I asked her what she wanted to do. I gave her three options; go somewhere grab coffee and talk, stay home and chat or go take pictures in the woods together and chat. No contest, we decided to take pictures in the woods.

I took her to the low ropes course by my old apartment complex I lived in with Nick to take pictures and go for a walk and talk. It was nice; sun was out; snow was clinging to the ground in the forest trails, a perfect late fall early winter day. We came to a bridge in the middle of the woods on a frozen swamp that I had run over many a day. I had to bring my engagement ring (long story) back from California to get it checked to keep the warranty on it, and for SOME reason... I put the ring in my pocket for the ride home. Can't store those things, expensive. Once we got to the bridge, I felt the ring and started to laugh a bit thinking about the 'hypothetical situation' of, "what if I asked her to marry me now?" Then I started to get nervous and laugh some more because I knew that I was going to ask her. Luckily, my mind thinks a million miles a minute, so I weighed the pros and cons of it all, and she was DEFINITELY worth it. She was everything I was looking for, and more, so why put it off? And dating sucks, especially long distance dating with somebody you don't know all the details about. It becomes a bunch of 'dating games' mixed with an inability to talk about the important stuff you both want to work towards and a side of "do I really want to invest the time, effort and money into this relationship if there's a chance it might not work out".

And if you think about it, dating is basically staying with that person until you feel they're not good enough for you and then you leave. It can be very selfish; it's like practicing for divorce! One of my favorite quotes from my good friend Bill Hastings, "*$@% the details! Leave the little things to little people, focus on the big picture." Okay, I'll get off my soapbox now.

From there I told her that she is an absolutely amazing woman, and I might not know all the little details about her, but I know the more important things about her and I wanted to spend the rest of my life with her. Then I got down on one knee and asked her to marry me while pulling the ring out of the pocket and displaying it. My knee got wet. But more importantly, she said yes! I can't believe she said yes! Crazy. I guess you could say I asked her to marry me on our first date. Granted, the first date may have been a few day experience, but I guess I can still say it. Then I told the family, and they were shocked… and then they weren't shocked… and then they were happy… and then Uncle Joe was impressed. I appreciated that the most. I'm not sure why, maybe just that he agreed with it so much, but understood how hard it must have been to do something like that. Who knows. Cam was the least surprised… obviously. The funny thing was, is that I was actually surprised too while it was happening. Not saying it was out of character completely for me, but it's definitely something I didn't foresee coming I guess. But I'm sure I wasn't as surprised as she was.

Then it was time to meet the parents; she's from Frederick, South Dakota. South Dakota is FA-REEZING in December! I came out the next weekend to meet them and was met with a blizzard and some very cold weather. I was not prepared for this kind of weather. It reminded me all over again of why I moved from Michigan to California. It was hard to train over there, but Northern State University let me in on their indoor track so I was able to do some repeats on their track. But for some of my other workouts, I had to run for five to ten minutes, go back in her apartment, do some pushups, sit ups, dips and arm curls, then start running again after I warmed up.

I was running once while Kelsea was at basketball practice at Northern University in Aberdeen, and I had to go into their sports complex to get out of the cold. I was having the same problems I had the year before in Michigan, couldn't run much more than ten minutes. Luckily, the Northern Cross Country team was getting ready to go out for a run, so I decided to run with them. It's amazing how much easier it is to run in freezing cold conditions with a team. I made it about eight miles straight with them, furthest I got all winter in South Dakota.

But I distinctly remember one run where I had to run about half a mile with that wind to the main road that was fine; but then I had to run south for about two minutes, then switch and run north for two minutes when one side of my face was frozen from the wind and cold. The only thing that kept me going was waiting for Kelsea to drive by from Basketball Practice to pick me up. If she didn't, I would have to jog a little over a quarter mile into the 40 MPH head wind with golf ball sized snow flakes to get back to her house. If that would happen, I would cry. If I cried it would freeze, and then I would cry more. Vicious cycle. It was hard to see through the wind and snow, but I did make out her car coming at me. I started to wave fanatically and jump around like a maniac. She waved at me and drove on by… dang it. I had to run the long quarter mile back. I ran it all backwards though, so it wasn't completely awful, just awkward. I got back and we had our first fight. Okay, we really didn't fight, but I did have an urge to throw a snowball at her.

She has an awesome family and that made it easy to come in and say, "Hey… yeah, I'm the crazy guy that asked your daughter to marry me the first time we met." I didn't really say that, but it was implied. And for a little town of only 250 people, they have an amazing high school gym and workout facility! If you're ever in Fredrick, South Dakota, go to their high school and work out there, it's awesome. I had a great time there with their family and also with their shotguns, pheasants, buffalo, and elk. If you ever want to go for a buffalo or 60 point elk hunt give her dad, Randy Barondeau, a call in Fredrick, South Dakota. I will get mine some day.

I continued with my training plan during and after that trip. Back in California, I had one run where there were 100 mph gusts in the mountains nearby and 60 mph gusts where I was running with HUGE drops of rain coming down practically sideways. I thought to myself, "it's not cold, I can run in this." And I went for a run in that weather. I actually saw trees and large branches coming down around me and I'll admit, I was a little scared. I thought about going into my club or a gas station or something nearby, but because it was kind of cold and wet out, I was wearing full body spandex and I looked like a scuba diver. I do have a little pride, at least enough to prevail against physical wellbeing.

I ran with the wind the first three miles out. That was stupid. The second and third miles were around 4:30 mile pace, but on a normal day they would have been around 5:30 mile pace. Coming back took a bit longer, and the rain REALLY hurt. I had to run with my hand over my eyes the whole way back. Luckily, nobody could really see me through the rain or that my hand was covering my face or they probably would have thought I was an idiot. I fooled them all.

I returned to South Dakota to spend Christmas with the new family. Then I brought her whole family back to Michigan with me for New Years! After that, I flew her out to see me in California in late January. There were many hours in planes traveling and heaps of social energy used in those couple of months there, but training was still going great! It might have been because of the excitement of it all, but I was feeling pretty good. I was pretty busy at this time, I was still coaching a few high school 800 meter guys, I started selling Cutco Knifes (which I found out takes more time than they lead you to believe), I was personal training nine clients, talking to Kelsea for hours a night (which I enjoyed immensely), and of course training my butt off. Goooo unsponsored athlete's crazy lives!

I decided to run the University of Washington Invite to try out my new taper for the first time. I call it "My Completely Shererious Taper". I just made that up. But I really like it. Anyways, I trained hard for a couple weeks, followed by four days easy, and then started my very hard training sequence approximately one week away from my race. I ran an 800 and a 400 at Willie's "Los Gatos All Comer Meet" the Saturday before the meet. I ran a 1:52 in the 800 and a 50.5 for the 400 meter.

Kelsea was there to cheer me on to victory. I romped all over some high schoolers. So in good sportsmen like behavior, I ran backwards for the last 10 meters and point right at them. Just kidding, I didn't point or run backwards at all... I gave them high fives as they crossed the line.

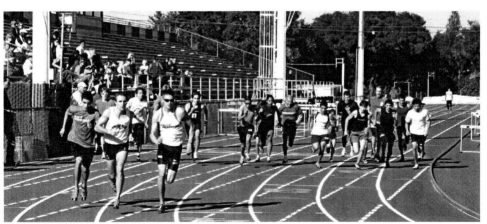

Kian Banks, Tim Bayley, me   lil' tikes

Los Gatos All-Comers Meet: 800 Start   Photo by: Jerry Banks

The next day, Sunday, I ran a hill interval workout and lifted with my legs heavily. On Monday I ran five miles in 25:06 with Kelsea biking beside me in the rain and then also did a hard Navy Seal Upper body workout. On Tuesday, I did 8 x 400 in about 60 seconds with one minute rest in-between. On Wednesday, I ran another shorter tempo and an easy shake out run. Then on Friday I did 10 x 200 starting at a 27 and ended in 25's with as much rest as I wanted between each one. On Thursday, the day before my big opener, I took really easy. I did two runs of about twelve minutes going about ten minute pace per mile. I actually really do go that slowly for recovery runs... I will jog a mile and you can time me! Then I did another really slow shake out run about five hours before my race. I couldn't tell if I felt good or not, I knew I was nervous. I spent a good amount of money on hotel and plane tickets and I didn't know if I was going to come up here and suck again like I did 2 years ago with the farm team! I mean, my taper had never been tested before; it could be crap for all I knew at this point. Luckily, it wasn't crap, far from it.

The warm up for my first indoor race was interesting, didn't really know how I felt. With the nerves of racing it's always hard to tell how I feel before a race. By the time I do my strides I have a good idea of how the race is going to go. I felt snappy and quick during my strides, which meant it was going to be good. I was excited, but still nervous. I decided I'd just go with the group and see what happened.

The start of my first mile race felt really slow to me and we were right at about 60 second pace for about 800 meters. Then with about 500 to go, I took off and ran a very fast lap to get the facility record, the world leading time, and the fastest mile ran indoor by an American in the last two years! I ran a 3:56.00 mile, over five seconds faster than my previous life time best I'd gotten four years before. It was nine seconds faster than I had ran the year before, and 21 seconds faster than I ran two years before on the same track. I was on cloud nine, I ran to my car and texted my whole phone.

I called Kelsea right away, but no answer, so I called my dad, he did. It was great, I was so happy I didn't even know what to do with myself, so I frolicked. Well actually, I just went for a brief cool down and thanked all the people congratulating me. I paced the 3k for a little over 2000 meters after that and it felt so easy. People have told me, I should have finished, but I decided not to. I actually didn't know if my time would count being the pacer, so didn't want to waste the race effort. After that I flew back home, still on cloud nine.

I got to the airport and found out I put AM instead of PM on my flight. So it had already taken off. Go figure. But I was having a good day and they let me go through on standby for the next flight at no extra charge, which was sweet. Then, things quickly went from good to great. After talking to some friends and family who were calling me on the phone and congratulating me on the race, the flight desk people called my name. I went up there and they told me that I got on the flight! I was still ecstatic about my race so I said, "Thank you so much! Things have been going amazing today! I ran a mile today at University of Washington and now I'm the fastest miler in the world this year!" I think I put it so it sounded like a bigger deal than it was, but it was good enough. She said, "Well then let's put you in first class!" I thought it was a good call. So I got on the plane, and I'm riding with the entire Stanford Men's and Woman's Track and Field team, and the entire Stanford Men's and Woman's Basketball team! The lady from the desk came on the plane and told the stewardess that I was the fastest miler in the world, so she announced it to the entire plane. Then the whole plane of Stanford Athletes clapped for me!

As awkward as that was, it was pretty stinkin' sweet! I sat with a really tall Stanford Basketball player named Josh Owens in first class. That was nice, he's a cool guy. The stewardess also kept bringing me wine and asking me about running. Then after Josh stopped chatting, I decided to watch some stand-up comedians on my computer. Let me tell you, there is no better way to fly than a few wines down, in first class and watching stand-up comedians with the whole plane of Stanford Athletes cheering for you. I didn't want to land!

Soon enough, however, we did end up landing. I was okay with that; had some things to do. I got into the Tyson Invite at Arkansas. Ray Flynn helped me out with that a little bit. That the race was coming up with not much down time between races. I had to figure out how to use my taper and still train hard to get in better shape in two weeks. So I did the same exact thing for the most part. I always switch up my workouts a little bit depending on how I'm feeling, but it was as close as I could get it. I felt really good there, but I wanted to run much faster than the pace we were going. I took off a little early this time, with about 600 plus to go. Nick Willis went right with me; good ol' roomy. He has a better kick than I do, so he took off at 300 to go and I tried my best to stay with him, but that guy can make 50 second pace look like a jog at the end of a race. He's efficient. He won the race and Sullivan got me too, but I still got a decent time there. It was nice to see Nick again too, if you don't know him you should. I recommend a Nick Willis for everybody. Kidding, but he is a great person.

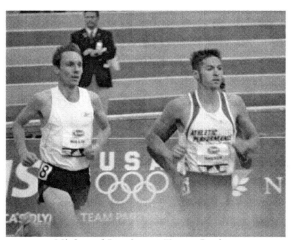
Nick and I racing at Tyson Invite

After that I only had one week to do my taper! I was kind of at a loss as to how to do it, but I decided to take a couple days easier and then do the same thing going into nationals. I'm pretty sure it worked, however, my race strategy did not. I decided to go to the back to stay out of trouble thinking it'd be a slow tactical race.

Unfortunately, it was not. Somebody had planted a rabbit in the race and it went out fast. I was ok with it, but I just waited a little bit too long to make my move. I went from the back of the pack to try and get in the lead with about 400 to go. I was moving really fast in lane three around the corner and then I met Will Leer's back as he was falling to the ground. Luckily for him, I had to push him forward to not trip over him, and he shot forward. Unluckily for me I lost all my momentum for the backstretch. I tried to pass Rob with 300 to go, but that guy has one mean kick too, and I could get around him. I tried to tuck in behind him for the curve but I met Russell Brown there so I moved in behind him. I tried a couple more times to pass them but they matched my moves well. I had lost all my kick in the corner collision. I shouldn't have let myself get into trouble that late in a race, but you can't account for every-thing either. It was still a big disappointment; I really wanted to make a team very badly.

I still had the Olympic Trials to look forward to, and that was my new focus. It seemed like a feasible goal since I had been rocking indoor. I didn't take that much time off from indoors and really started right up for outdoors again. The Stanford Invite was in a few weeks so I figured I'd train right up until that and see what I could do. I decided to run the 800 to open up in the outdoor sea-son. I thought I could run a 1:47 for an opener, maybe even 1:46 if I was on my A game. A few days before the race I rolled my ankle really good on a tempo run. I jogged it off but my knee was more soar than my ankle after that. I didn't think too much of it because I have had knee problems before and this was nothing compared to that pain. But I guess I SHOULD have thought more of it because I've had knee problems. I got to the race a couple days later and I could still feel it, but nothing serious.

I ran the race and didn't feel it at all, must have been the adrena-line. I went a little too late for a fast time. I sat right in the back of the pack until about 250 to go and took off to try and get the lead from the back. I moved to the front pack pretty easily but then I couldn't get around Kevin Hicks, so I ran along his shoulder. I had learned from indoors not to try and tuck back in, it doesn't happen if you hesitate. I still couldn't get around him for the win, but I still ran 1:48 low, so it was a pretty good opener for me. I felt really good the whole way, but I came through a little too slow at 400 to get a really good time. I should have moved up earlier, but I hesitated to move up that soon because I wasn't sure of myself yet being the first outdoor race. I decided to run the 1500 the next day, but this didn't go well at all. I took the lead at 400 and tried to keep a good pace. But something wasn't right, maybe it was the 800 from the day before, but I didn't think that was it. I came through 1200 at around 2:58 or so and then the whole pack passed me like a wave at 200 to go. I tried to go with them but I was tying up bad. I crossed the line in 3:45. Not a good opener for outdoors and my knee was hurting afterwards, double dang.

I decided to do a hill repeat workout the next day since I felt like I didn't do much on the Stanford track the day before. This was a bad idea. My nagging knee wasn't too bad enough at this point, but it soon would be. I ran my patented hill repeat workout but had to walk down for most of the mountain. For some reason, I still didn't even think much about it. I figured my knee was just a little soar from the hills, but that it would go away. Nope, I was wrong, the knee pain stayed. I still have no idea what it was, but it was a deep sharp pain on my outside knee right where the IT band attaches to the knee. The next day I couldn't even run ten feet without excruciating knee pain.

People tend to think the worse about something like this, and I was no exception. I thought I had a micro tear in my ACL, or something like that, and I might have made it worse by running on it. I was freaking out; I thought I had ruined my Olympic hopes by doing something stupid. My goal was to try and get there out of pure intelligent training, and this didn't look good on the resume. I tried everything to get better: knee wraps, IT band strength routines, stretching, hot-cold treatment, heating creams, tons of glucosamine, chondroitin, MSM and fish oil. But nothing helped that much at all. I couldn't even aqua jog to cross train because it bent my knee and made it really soar after five minutes or less. I was pretty worried. Since I couldn't do anything for cross training, I thought my fitness was going to head out the window. I was scared.

Just less than three weeks went by and I still couldn't even jog. I had signed up to do the Drake Relays and I really wanted to go because I had never gone before. They were also giving me an appearance fee, which I had never gotten before. I decided it was now or never and I went to the track, put on my spikes, barely did anything except leg swings to warm up, and did a 400 around the track around 60 second pace. My knee felt tolerable, so I tried it again. I went a little quicker this time, and with no pain! So I waited a minute and gave it another shot. My lungs started to feel it, but my legs were still ok. I did a couple more before I'd had enough and I was pretty excited to say the least! I couldn't cool down because my knee pain came back, but at least I could handle the faster paces again! I had tried this earlier in my injury period and it didn't work at all. After this workout, I decided to go to Drake. I hadn't done any workouts, running, or anything except for this one 400-meter workout in three weeks, but I sort of hoped it'd be like a serious taper. I hopped on the plane and took off for Drake.

Drake was a great experience. There was a ton of people I knew from Belgium and Nationals there to race, so I had a good time hanging out with some cool athletes like Nikeya Green, Toyin Augustus and some other sprinters I had the pleasure to meet. They treated us like royalty there. If you ever have a chance to run there, do it! It's a very well put on meet. The hotel they put us in was really nice as well. I had a room all to myself with a bag full of goodies; life was good.

I had a good time except for my race. Luckily it was windy so they took it out a little slower and I had no problems for the first 1200 meters. I felt so good I decided to take over the lead, so I shot to the front. This might have been a bad move, because I ran out of gas at about 200 to go. I called a friend to drop off a gallon of gas for me, but no dice! I was on my own. I tried to close with the guys but had no closing speed; I ran a 4:09 outdoor mile. I would have been kind of embarrassed about it, but the winner was only 4:05 because of the wind, so at least I was within rocks throw of the winner. He's lucky I didn't bring my throwing rock. Actually, be-lieve it or not; I do not have currently own a throwing rock yet, I'll have to look on E-bay. After the race, I tried to cool down with Matt Gabrielson, but I only made it like a mile and a half. But on the plus side, that was the furthest I'd been able to jog in over three weeks! So I was happy about the jog at a brisk pace.

The next big race for me was a road mile. I had never raced a road mile before, but this was kind of a great opportunity. There was some prize money on the table for this race, they paid for my trip over there, and more importantly, they paid for my trip to my wedding! That was nice of them. The Medtronic TC 1 Mile was on the 8th of May in Minneapolis, Minnesota, and I was getting married on the 10th of May in Aberdeen, South Dakota. I was cutting it close, but I like to live on the edge. I still couldn't train that much in between the last race and this one because of my knee. I had to depend on my high quality workouts with pretty much no base runs. I ran an alright road mile, but I still had no endurance at all. The last 300 meters of the race I faded a bit. I got riz-ocked. But I ended up doing a fartlek afterwards at night in the park for 40 minutes and I felt really good! No knee pain at all! I was stoked. I could feel it before the race, and then I didn't feel it anymore for the rest of the season. I had not been able to run for over ten minutes before this race. I had still been able to do a few track workouts for some weird reason, which didn't make any sense! But this seemed to be the abrupt end of my knee injury. Maybe I was so excited to get married my brain didn't register the pain anymore. I recom-mend marriage to everybody, definitely worth it!!

Most of my wedding party flew in to South Dakota before me since I had to fly in the next day; the day before the wedding. It was an amazing wedding, probably the best ever recorded in the history of weddings. The only way it could have been topped is if we in-cluded my brilliant idea of having my groomsmen and I swinging in from the rafters with old bushy armed pirate-like Victorian shirts on. That didn't happen, so that was the only bad part. Waiting for the gun to go off in a track race had nothing on waiting for my soon-to-be wife to walk down that isle. Funny thing was that this time I really couldn't lose like in a race! But I was still very nervous to say the least.

Just two days after the wedding, Kelsea and I drove right back to California. We made it in a straight shot too, and it was a long drive. We left at 3:00 in the morning from South Dakota and arrived in California the next day at 3:45 in the morning. There was a two hour time change as well, so we definitely slept in. That was sort of our temporary honeymoon for the time being; I couldn't take a long break from running because I had to get ready for the Olympic Trials in a month and some change. But I was really glad she was there to help me out in life… it's not easy sometimes.

After the wedding, I had zero knee pain and I could finally train like I wanted to train. I still avoided hills awhile after the wedding though, just to be sure. I did a low-key race in Southern California; I won the 800 and felt good. But it was really cold and windy so I only ran a 1:50. I decided to hop in the 1500 for a workout; I wanted to get something out of driving all the way down there to race. But I had lost all my endurance for a 1500 so I faded again at 300 to go and only ran a hard 3:45. I was heading in the right direction, but not fast enough. I only had a 3:41.0 to my name thus far and I wasn't sure that would get me into the trials. I figured I'd get it done at Occidental where I always got it done before; the Jim Bush Invitational.

I felt really ready for this one, training was really coming around finally and I was really excited to race. I got a hotel online and did my 200 workout two days before and was feeling great and fast. The next day I was driving down and my Dad called and asked if I was at the meet. I said, "PSSSSSSHHHHH!!! Come on Dad, its tomorrow!" He then told me that all the websites he looked at told him it was today. I was a little worried, but still confident that it was the next day on Sunday. Jim Bush had always been on the first Sunday in June, so I called my buddy Tim Bayley who was going to the meet just to make sure I was right. He picked up the phone and said, "Ello Mate! Ya here?!" (He's British) I said, "Not yet, isn't the meet tomorrow?" He said, "No it's today, we're all here in the hotel waiting to go over." So I said, "Well craptabulous! I'll be there ASAP." I still had about a four and a half hour drive to get to the meet. Luckily, I had a wife to help bail me out of a sticky situation. I asked her to drive so my legs would be a little fresher, and she agreed. Unfortunately, I put myself back into a sticky situation and spilled hot coffee all over myself. There was nothing she could do about that one, she was driving.

We got there and still had about an hour and a half before the race. I tried to wash the coffee off of me and relax a second before I warmed up. I decided to run the 800; I really wanted to get the A standard because I figured I'd have a much better shot at making a team in the 800. I tried not to think of the workout I did the day before, the long car ride here and the coffee smell coming from my body. Luckily it all went away when I realized I forgot my Jersey and had nothing to run in. Fortunately, people kept bailing me out of my own lack of preparation. My buddy Rob Mandje let me borrow his jersey for the race. It was a nice jersey too, he's lucky he got it back.

After I warmed up and stepped on the line. I didn't think anybody was going to take the lead for the first lap. If they didn't, then it'd be hard to run a fast time without any help after a day like mine. I was right; I had to lead it in a 53 second first lap. I didn't really think I could do another one by myself so I stepped off the track. I had signed up for the 1500 and that had more depth in the race and it also had a couple of rabbits. Luckily, the meet was running behind schedule, and that gave me a little extra time to get ready for the race.

The race finally started and it was very well set up. We had a couple of rabbits take us through 800 meters at a solid pace. But it ended up being around 2 minutes for the 800. I felt pretty good so I went with 500 to go on the home stretch and took the lead. I pushed it as hard as I could to get a good time, and I got it. I ran another lifetime best of 3:40 to win the race. I was mainly happy that I didn't waste a trip down there, especially with how the day had been going. I was fairly confident 3:40 would get me into the trials. And that was 'very positive' as they say in Vector Marketing.

There was a race in Cambridge, Canada for a Mercedes Benz, and they would pay for a flight for Kelsea and me to get there. This was fairly close to my parents' house so I figured it was a free flight home! I always like coming home, so I really wanted to race there. The only thing was that this was a big racing weekend and I still wanted to get a better time in the 800 and the 1500. The mile in Cambridge wouldn't count for anything, but the winner would receive a new Mercedes Benz. And I'm not in it for the money, cars, fame and women; I'm in it for the free bananas after the race. Ok I'm not, plus most races don't provide bananas for me after the meet. There was an American Milers Club series down in Indianapolis, IN that had a few good mid-distance races going on that week, so I decided to drive down on Wednesday and try to get the 800 A standard. I knew from my workouts that I was in shape to do it; I just had to get in the right race. I saw some big names in the race, so I was excited. My parents were nice enough to drive Kelsea and me the five-hour trip down there in the back of their minivan. After getting lost a few times on the 'scenic' route, we made it down there. I got ready for the race and then heard they put me in the slow section... with no rabbit. I was pretty upset that I had made my parents drive me down here and everything to get into the slow section of the 800. There were guys in the fast section that probably would have done better in our heat. But I held it together; I didn't flip out and steal a goldfish or anything. I tried to focus on my race and running it fast.

My start in the 800 normally isn't the greatest, so I didn't get out very good in the first 200 meters. Then the next 200 slowed down a little bit, but I went at 400 because it was a little slow again. Running in lane two sucks on the curve for the 800, I don't recommend it at all. I finally took the lead at 300 to go and tried to keep picking it up as much as possible. I held on for the win and went 1:47.9 again, but that wouldn't get me into the trials. The fast race was won in 1:45, I know I could have been in that race for the win if I was in it. Oh well, I did like the meet and the race conditions were perfect on a pretty hard track surface, so I thought about coming back down for the Saturday meet. However, it was still a long car ride back.

The only problem was that I was planning on racing in Cambridge that Saturday evening. After much consideration, I finally decided to run the meet in Indy. I entered in the 800, but everybody was trying to convince me to run the 1500. It was a tough call, both were going to be fast races, and I was guaranteed into both fast heats this time. The 1500 was going to be paced by Alan Webb, so I figured the pacing would be perfect. But I really wanted the 800 time for the trials. After talking to my Agent Ray Flynn and my parents I decided to just run the 1500 and go for a really good time.

I drove myself down to Indy with Kelsea and got to the race well before race time. It was kind of funny to see that many amazing track athletes running and to have only a few fans there. I had a blast watching all the other races; I guess I'd figured there'd be more people there to enjoy the amazing display of talent. My race went just as I thought it would, fast.

It was a perfect night for good times in Indianapolis again, there was no wind, not too hot or too cold and I had dragged a beautiful woman out there to try and impress. There was about six guys all going for the A-standard in that race, so I had plenty of people to run with. It was a perfectly smooth race, we just all hoped on the rail and hung on to the quick pace. These are my favorite kind of races, everybody wants to go fast and you have a pacer to make sure it goes out fast, no bumping, shoving or spiking. The first rabbit dropped out at 600 and Webb took it the rest of the way to 1200 perfectly. He came through at around 2:53 with Nate Brannen and Chris Lukezic right on his tail. I was right behind them. It was painful to come through that fast, but I wasn't dead by a long shot. I did sort of hesitate going at that point thinking it might be too early or they would pick it up themselves; so I waited till 100 to go. I took off and stayed as smooth as possible running as fast as I could to cross the line first in 3:36.81; a monster PB for me. I was ecstatic all over again! I was finally back and even better than indoors! The rest of the night was spent talking to friends and family and driving home. It was a good drive back this time.

At that point in the year, there were only three other Americans who had run faster than me that year. I thought my chances at the trials were all right. Good thing I didn't know I had to get the A-standard at or before the trials to go to the Olympics in Beijing, or that would have really ruined my happiness. Especially being only .2 away from the A Standard. Every other National Championship or Olympic Trials before this one the athlete could just compete at the trials, and then go for the A-standard in Europe after the trials if he hadn't gotten it already. I knew running without the A-standard would be like running with my shoes tied together, blind folded and my hands tied behind my back. I almost went to the line at the trials like that in protest, but opted not to at the last minute.

I went up to Eugene, Oregon, a little early for the trials; there had been about 300 forest fires in northern Cali at the time, which made the air quality awful. I didn't want this to give me breathing problems or flare up my asthma so I decided to go to Eugene early. Good choice, they had a waffle machine for breakfast at every hotel we stayed at. But they also had forest fire smoke for the few extra days I stayed there as well. For some reason it's hard to eat the few days before big meets like this. I think the nerves of the race make you queasy and not hungry. I think if I didn't get my mind off of the race I could have died from nerve poisoning before the race.

Kevin helped me out again, he let me stay at his place after he was done racing. Kelsea's parents came up to watch me race and my parents did as well. I wish I could have been more entertaining, but the nerves paralyzed me the whole weekend. Some people say they don't like racing because of all the nerves, and I can totally understand and relate to that feeling. However, I love nerves; it's a rush that some people just can't take. Like peering off that 65ft high cliff, or waiting for my future wife to walk down that isle. The feelings were pretty similar for the couple days cooped up in a hotel room before the trials. The main difference was that I had to experience these racing nerves for almost a week straight. Sometimes it's not good to stay in that nervous excitement state for long periods of time, so I did everything I could to get rid of it for now… then embrace those nerves like a lost puppy for race day.

Race day was the worst of all the nerve days. I had never raced well at a National Championship event. I seem to enjoy racing stupid and miss making it to the finals; last year I was dead last! The first race was the most nerve raking for me. I decided to not go out in 55 seconds for my first lap like I did last time; actually I went right to the back of the pack. I chose the Nick Willis Style of championship racing; go to the back for the first two laps, then move to the front and take off with 400 or less to go. It worked. I moved to the front on the home stretch with 500 to go. I sat there running comfortably equal to the other runner in the lead. It was pretty amazing to be in the lead at the Olympic trials, feeling really good, hearing the bell for the final lap and the crowd's cheers start to get louder... I soaked it all in. At 300 hundred to go I started to pick it up to make sure I was top six and wasn't out kicked by a bunch of short kickers with 50 to go. I knew I was in for sure at 200 to go, I could hear people behind me, but I was feeling like I had another gear if I had to use it. All I had to do was get top six, so I kept the pace but relaxed as much as possible to save some for the next day. Then, a race savvy Gabe Jennings decided to kicked me down the last ten meters, which gave me a comfortable second place.

This was a huge accomplishment for me; it calmed me down a little for the next couple races. The hard one was out of the way, I had my confidence back. The nerves were still there, not as killer as the previous couple of days, but it was definitely there the whole night and next day.

The next race I did the same thing, since it worked so well before. The race went out a little quicker than before, but sort of clumped back up at 600 meters in. I decided to move to the shoulder of the leader at 800 from the back and take off at a lap to go. I went to the shoulder and Webb picked it up. This gave me a perfect spot right behind him. I decided to just sit there unless somebody tried to pass me. Rob decided he wanted to pass me, and he did with a little more than a 100 to go, so I went with him. Finished in fourth overall because of Legat and Leers quick last 20 meters, but I was just going for top six so I wasn't worried too much near the finish. If you want a little more detail for this race, go back and read the intro again.

I was in the finals, and it was game time. Now I was seriously nervous. I thought I had a chance to go, but I still needed the A-standard along with half the other runners in the race. I had no idea what to do for the finals. This is where a coach would have been nice to have; somebody to tell me what to do so I didn't have to drive myself crazy thinking about what to do with all the million and one different ways the race could turn out. I had a whole day to think myself into the dirt about the race. I still felt good, no soreness at all from the previous races. The only thing on my mind was how the race was going to go out. I was hoping that somebody would take it out fast from the gun and it would be a "whoever is the fastest will win" type of race. But the only one in that race strong enough to do it was not in top shape yet. Alan Webb took it from the gun last year and looked really good while doing it. I hoped he would do it again, but I kind of doubted it. The only other person that could take it from the gun was Benard Lagat, but he never goes fast before 200 to go; I kind of doubted he'd do it now. Manzano and Lemong had run fast, but never by themselves. Another factor… that turned into a big factor was the wind that decided to pick up near the race.

We all got to the line; the last race of the Olympic Trials. The scene was fantastic; they really did a great job for the trials in Eugene. The stands were packed, the announcer was blaring and the crowd was roaring. Watching the finals of the 800 a week before was amazing. I had never heard a louder track crowd before in my life and never wanted to be in a race as much as I wanted to be in that one either. It was all very cool, and now it was my time to race. I was hoping they would get out fast and I could get in the top pack on a line. This did not happen. Legat stormed out to the front and slammed on the breaks to slow the whole race down. This effectively ruined the race for half of the athletes that didn't have the standard. It also made the whole pack run into each other so the whole first lap was a shove fest. I don't like being pushed, it destroys your concentration on the race and makes it near impossible to relax. If I can't relax in a race it doesn't matter how slow we go out my lungs close up on me. And that's exactly what happened to me. With two laps to go I could feel my lungs starting to shrink and I knew the race was over. You can't run fast without oxygen and I've proved that theory many a time. I was actually in good position for the kick, but I couldn't go any faster without oxygen. I tried as hard as I could to relax my lungs and body, but it didn't help at all.

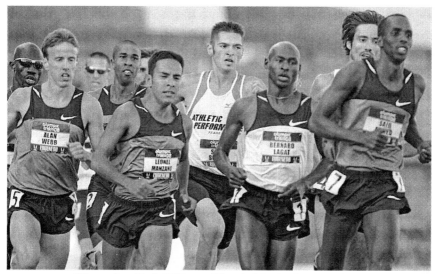

Photo by: *Bob Elliott, The Athletic Connection*

After the race people tried to interview me, but I was so oxygen deprived I barely even remember it. I was hanging from the fence, laying on the ground, my head was pounding, felt like I was going to vomit and I'm pretty sure all the color in my face was gone. But I wanted to be nice and answer the questions they had for me. Interviewers, "Steve, how was the race?" Me, "Close to as bad as I look right now..." After that I couldn't get off my back in the changing tent. They told me they were going to get a cart if I couldn't get up; so I got up, walked outside the tent, went out of sight of the staff on the side of the tent and then proceeded to lie back down. The staff girl walked out of the tent and found me out there... she called for a cart. First time I have ever been carted off from a race before, but man did I feel awful.

They got me to the medical tent (I was the only one there the whole day they told me), and then I finally threw up. It's amazing how much better you feel after getting that crap out of your system. I finally got up and started walking back to the hotel. Kelsea and the family had already walked back to the hotel. I guess I was there for a long time, I really had no idea.

That was kind of the end of my storybook season. Didn't end with a Cinderella story appearance into the Olympic games, but it does end in determination. I have learned a great deal over the last two years and am still learning. I do not have it all figured out but I feel I am getting close, and I will keep improving. This year I learned more than I have about running my entire career of running, and I won't sit and stagnate on that juicy piece of information, but will try to build upon that information and make it even better.

Since I started coaching myself I have learned that I need to keep learning and then improving on what I know works for me. The minute you think you have it all figured out and this is as good as it will get, you'd better have already gotten some records and made some teams, because if you always do what you've always done you'll always get what you've always got. That's what makes America great, if you find a better way to do something it's celebrated. In some countries that don't appreciate differences there is a saying, "the nail that sticks out gets the hammer", but Americans appreciate innovators. And now you know a different way to build a program and can take some tools from my tool chest and add them to your own. Hopefully they work as well for you as they have for me.

Take what you want out of this book to enhance your training, leave the rest, and enjoy the process. Then perhaps someday you can write a detailed book about how you broke numerous barriers in your life to help other curious people out of a training rut. Keep training hard and enjoy the process!

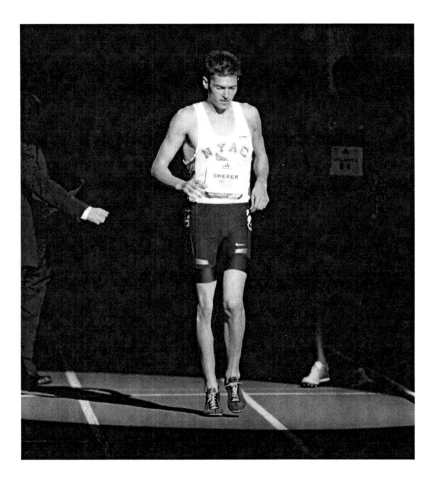

Photo by: *Bob Elliott, The Athletic Connection*

"If you can make yourself enjoy pushing your body as hard as it can go until you achieve complete muscle fatigue, imagine how much fun the rest of your life will be!" ~ Steve Sherer

Offramp720@gmail.com

steve shererl@gmail.com

LaVergne, TN USA
27 September 2009

159115LV00004B/117/P